ECGs FOR HE
PROFESSIONALS

Han B Xiao MD PhD
Consultant Cardiologist, Homerton Hospital, London

Henry Purcell MB PhD
Senior Fellow in Cardiology, Royal Brompton Hospital, London

Rubin Minhas MB BCh
General Practitioner, and CHD Lead, Medway Primary Care Trust, Kent

Published by Concise Clinical Consulting
48 Old Church Street, London SW3 5BY
© Concise Clinical Consulting 2007

The right of Han B Xiao, Henry Purcell and Rubin Minhas to be identified as authors of this work has been asserted by them in accordance with the Copyright, Designs and Patents Act 1988.

ISBN: 978-0-9555454-0-5

British Library Cataloguing-in-Publication Data
A catalogue record for this book is available from The British Library

Note:
Medical knowledge is constantly changing. As new information becomes available, changes in treatment, procedures, equipment and the use of drugs becomes necessary. The editors/authors/contributors and the publishers have taken care to ensure that the information given in this text is accurate and up to date. However, readers are strongly advised to confirm that the information, especially with regard to drug usage, complies with the latest legislation and standards of practice.

Design and layout production:
Consultants in Design
2 Pentlow Street, London SW15 1LX

Printed by: Printwright

CONTENTS

ACKNOWLEDGEMENTS

The editors are indebted to colleagues at
The Central Middlesex Hospital and Ealing
Hospital, London, particularly Ms Clare Turner
and Ms Leah Middlemas, both Cardiac
Technicians at Ealing Hospital, who recorded
and collected many of the ECGs in this book.

PART 1
BASICS OF
ELECTROCARDIOGRAPHY

01 INTRODUCTION

The electrocardiogram (ECG) is a thing of mystery to many. It need not be. While there is a wealth of science and understanding behind recording the electrical activity of the heart, in practice, much of the interpretation of what's going on is a matter of familiarity and pattern recognition. The aim of this book is to make things as uncomplicated as possible, not to explain the background science but to provide readers with simple guide to the ECG.

In this age of the Quality and Outcomes Framework (QOF), it is increasingly important to target patients at high risk of cardiovascular disease, i.e. those with severe hypertension, angina, heart failure and atrial fibrillation (AF). In other words, conditions likely to affect many of the elderly population. Of course, these problems are not exclusive to older people. The target organ damage of uncontrolled high blood pressure is seen in younger patients, too. All the more vital then, that we look for ECG tell-tale signs of left ventricular hypertrophy (LVH), which increases risk of stroke and sudden cardiac death, and needs aggressive antihypertensive treatment.

A study conducted among around 100 Merseyside general practitioners (GPs) in the early 1990s, showed that over 80% could identify a normal ECG. About one to two thirds correctly identified acute transmural ischaemia/infarction, but only 8-30% could accurately identify the site of the infarction and about a quarter of the GPs correctly interpreted non-acute abnormalities. The study suggested that a refresher course was warranted if these GPs were to be able to make a reliable diagnosis and give prehospital thrombolysis.[1] It is not only GPs who have difficulty reading ECGs. Another study[2] among hospital doctors showed that 74% could not accurately measure the PR interval.

Does this matter these days when we have rapid access chest pain clinics and automatic (interpretative) external defibrillators? Well, yes, it does. Everyone caring for patients would have some responsibility to diagnose correctly an acute coronary syndrome (for example). Likewise, basic distinction between atrial and ventricular tachyarrhythmias, and different types of heart block, could be critically important.

We encourage all those in the practice, therefore, to take time to systematically go through this little book. Learn to recognise the major ECG patterns and what they mean. Find out what to look for in an ECG machine, how to properly place the ECG leads and how to use the correct paper speed! But, most of all, enjoy the learning process.

REFERENCES

1   McCrea WA, Saltissi S. Electrocardiogram interpretation in general practice:relevance to prehospital thrombolysis. *Br Heart J* 1993;**70**:219-25.

2   Montgomery H, Hunter S, Morris S, Naunton-Morgan R, Marshall RM. Interpretation of electrocardiograms by doctors. *BMJ* 1994;**309**:1551-2.

02 ELECTRICAL ACTIVITY AND THE HEART

The electrical activity can be recorded from the outside (epicardium) or inside (endocardium) of the cardiac chambers, as well as the body surface, i.e. standard 12-lead ECG. The ECG is a graphic record of the electrical potentials of the heart.

The electrical activation is initiated in the sinus node, spread radially in all directions at atrial level by the myocardium and to the ventricles via the conduction system. The electrical signal travels along the conduction tissue at a speed of 4 m/s, and at approximately 1 m/s through the myocardium, more rapidly along than across the fibres. The surface ECG at any instant represents the total electrical activity of the myocardium. Its voltage is small as the signals cancel one another out.

Electrical conduction in the atria occurs via the musculature. There is no inter- or intra-atrial conduction pathway analogous to the His-Purkinje system in the ventricles. At ventricular level, the earliest myocardium to be activated is around the central point of the anterior wall of the left ventricle close to the interventricular septum. Activation spreads from there to the apex, base, lateral and posterior walls. The apex is activated before the base; the left ventricular free wall later than the right, while the posterior wall is the last to be excited. This normal pattern of ventricular activation sequence depends on the excitation wave being distributed through the atrioventricular bundle, left and right bundle branches.

Although the body surface ECG is the reflection of cardiac vector - the direction of electrical forces of the heart - this book will not cover its details in order to simplify the subject.

A set of letters have been used to label the electrical activities of the myocardium (figure 2-1).

P wave: the atrial electrical activity (depolarisation). It is normally <2.5 mm (0.25 mV) in height and ≤120 ms in duration.

PR interval: the time from the start of atrial activity to that of the ventricles, representing the atrioventricular conduction time. It is measured from the onset of the P wave to that of the QRS complex. It is normally between 120 and 210 ms, varying slightly with heart rate.

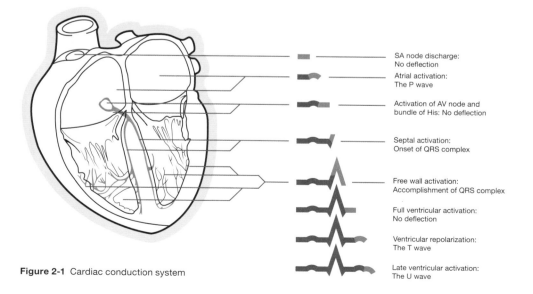

SA node discharge:
No deflection

Atrial activation:
The P wave

Activation of AV node and bundle of His: No deflection

Septal activation:
Onset of QRS complex

Free wall activation:
Accomplishment of QRS complex

Full ventricular activation:
No deflection

Ventricular repolarization:
The T wave

Late ventricular activation:
The U wave

Figure 2-1 Cardiac conduction system

PR segment: the time from the end of the P wave to the onset of the QRS complex. Its deviation may be evidence of atrial infarction.

QRS complex: the ventricular electrical signal. Q is the first negative deflection, R the first positive deflection, and S is the first negative deflection following a positive one. R' is the second positive deflection following a negative one. The QRS time interval is normally under 100 ms and QRS morphology varies with location where the record is made (see page 16).

QRS axis: usually referred to as the average direction of the ventricular electrical signal (vector). It is measured on the amplitude of the QRS complex in two (I and III) of the three standard limb leads. It is defined as the deviation from a horizontal line between the two arms of the individual (figure 2-2). When the QRS axis is normal, the dominant deflections are positive in both leads I and III. Left axis deviation is associated with dominant positive deflection in lead I and negative in lead III, and right axis deviation negative in lead I and positive in lead III.

ST segment: from the end of the QRS complex to the onset of the T wave. It is normally a horizontal line but may vary from -0.5 to +2 mm, particularly in chest leads.

T wave: the deflection produced by ventricular recovery. The direction of the T wave normally goes along with that of the QRS complex.

U wave: after or in the terminal portion of the T wave. It is normally small (<1/4 of T wave) and its exact genesis is unknown.

QT interval: the time from the onset of the QRS complex to the end of the T wave. QT interval varies with heart rate, empirically it is normally under half of the RR interval.

Sometimes corrected QT interval (QTc) is used. The concept of QTc is referred to the QT interval corrected for heart rate:

$$QTc = QT/\sqrt{RR} \text{ interval}$$

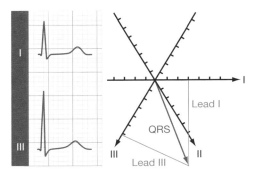

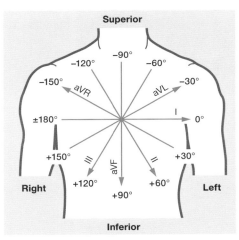

Figure 2-2 The simple method to assess the mean QRS axis is the triaxial reference system, where the three limb leads form 60° angles with each other and are divided into two halves, positive and negative from the centre. The algebraic sums of the amplitudes of the positive and negative waves in millimetres are calculated in leads I and III, and plotted on the corresponding axes. From the plotted points, perpendicular lines are dropped to a point of intersection. The line between the central point to the intersection represents the mean axis of the QRS complex.

In the same way, the mean axis of the P wave or the T wave can be calculated

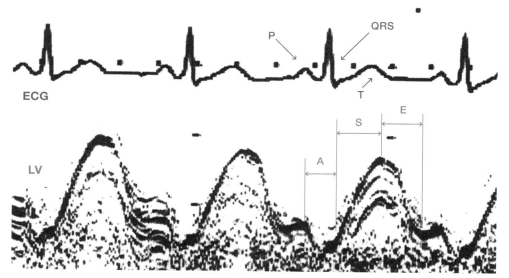

Figure 2-3 A simultaneous recording of the ECG and left ventricular (LV) longitudinal motion on M-mode echocardiography

Key: A: atrial contraction

S: left ventricular systole

E: left ventricular early diastole (early relaxation)

RR interval: the time between the peaks of two consecutive R waves. The heart rate can be calculated from the RR interval in two ways:

Heart rate = 60/RR interval (sec) or
Heart rate = 300/(number of big squares in one RR)

The atrial rate can be calculated in the same way from PP interval. In a normal heart, atrial and ventricular rates are identical. In patients with atrioventricular conduction disorder, atrial and ventricular rates differ and should be determined separately.

Generally speaking, the ECG deflections are markers of the mechanical cardiac cycle as the mechanical activities closely follow electrical signals. For example, atrial contraction (late diastole) follows P wave, ventricular contraction follows QRS complex and ventricular relaxation follows T wave. Figure 2-3 shows a more detailed account of this.

QUESTIONS & ANSWERS

1 How many small squares should accompany each of the components of the ECG waveforms?

A For P wave, there are 2 to 3 small squares; QRS complex, 2 to 2.5; PR interval 3 to 5. A simple way to calculate heart rate is to divide 300 by the number of boxes in the RR interval.

2 Many present day ECG machines provide interpretation. Does this mean that I do not need to understand the details of ECG waveforms?

A Automated ECG interpretation offers ECG diagnoses at a very high sensitivity in order to cover all possible abnormalities. It does not, however, indicate clinical relevance. Therefore it is best to understand the basics to be able to identify normal variations and recognise abnormal patterns, all of which are dependent upon a basic understanding of the ECG waveforms.

3 Are all elements of the ECG waveforms present in all patients?

A All elements of the ECG waveforms are certainly present in all normal subjects. But they vary greatly in patients - for instance, there may not be P waves in junction rhythm, there are less QRS complexes than P waves in complete heart block.

03 NORMAL ELECTROCARDIOGRAM

The most important first step towards clinical electrocardiography is to identify a normal electrocardiogram. This is not always easy, particularly when the clinical information is incomplete.

LEARNING POINTS

1   A normal ECG must be sinus rhythm and parameters in normal limits.

2   Dominant R wave in left sided-leads and dominant S wave in right-sided leads.

The basic normal ECG values are computer generated and shown in figure 3-1 (arrow).

A normal ECG has the following features:

1. Sinus rhythm characterised by a positive (upright) P wave in leads I, II, avF, V5 and V6, and a negative (downwards) P wave in avR and a biphasic one (positive then negative) in V1.

2. The heart rate is classically defined as between 50 and 100 beats/minute (bpm). We believe this should be re-assessed as it has been shown that there is an increased risk of cardiovascular events in people with resting heart rates over 80 bpm.

3. Every P wave is followed by a QRS complex. PR interval is between 120 and 200 ms. In leads I, avL, V5 and V6, there is a small q wave, which is the signal from the middle part of the ventricular septum and is thus referred to as the normal septal q wave.

   This septal q wave is 40 ms or less in time and a quarter or less in amplitude of the QRS complex. The total QRS duration is less than 100 ms. A QRS duration greater than 120 ms is termed as broad QRS complex and is a major feature of bundle branch block.

4. The mean QRS axis is between +10° and +90°, characterised by positive QRS complexes in both leads I and III.

5. The T wave is no less than 10% of the QRS complex in voltage and has the same direction as that of the QRS in the same lead. ST segment does not shift over 0.5 mm downwards or 1.5 mm upwards.

Even in a normal heart, the ECG waveforms vary greatly in different leads but follow a pattern:

Dominant R wave in left-sided leads, I, II, avL, V5 and V6

Dominant S wave in right-sided leads, avR, V1 and V2, which is the reflection of that from the left.

ECGs recorded in other leads (III, avF, V3 and V4) vary between the above two (figure 3-1).

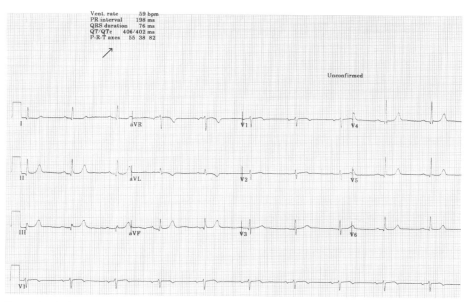

Figure 3-1 An ECG recorded in a normal subject. The traces in leads I, II, avL, V5 and V6 are nearly the mirror image of those in leads avR, V1 and V2

QUESTIONS & ANSWERS

1 Can patients with coronary artery disease have a normal ECG?

A Yes, certainly. As a matter of fact, the majority of patients with coronary artery disease may have a normal resting ECG. This is why those with suspected coronary artery disease have an exercise ECG to establish the diagnosis. In contrast, patients without coronary artery disease can have an abnormal ECG (there are a lot of cases in part II).

2 Do different ethnic populations have the same ECG?

A Yes, indeed. However, there is one particular variation in that young men of African origin are more likely to have a high voltage of the QRS complex and ST elevation without acute myocardial ischaemia.

3 In patients with a permanent pacemaker, does the ECG waveform differ from normal?

A Yes, the pacing ECG is significantly different from normal. The QRS complex is always wider than normal and there are abnormal ST-Ts in ventricular pacing, and P wave or PR interval is determined by the pacemaker (see part 2, chapter 19 for pacing ECG).

04 RECORDING TECHNIQUES

Both the interpretation and clinical value of an ECG are significantly affected by recording quality. Recognising artifacts is as important as diagnosing severe ECG abnormalities.

LEARNING POINTS

1   Recording quality is vital for interpretation.

2   Use the correct time and amplitude calibration.

3   An ECG is most commonly recorded by 12 standard leads.

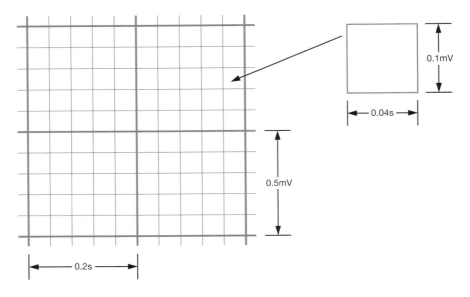

Figure 4-1 Illustration of time and amplitude scales of ECG recording paper

Recording paper

Normally, an ECG is recorded on specially designed graphic paper (figure 4-1), the vertical lines representing time and horizontal voltage. When the paper speed (or sweeping speed) is 25 mm/s, which is most commonly used, the distance between two thin vertical lines is 1 mm, representing 0.04 s (40 ms), while the interval between two thick lines is 5 mm, representing 0.2 s (200 ms). Today's ECG machines record digitally and print out so that measurements are made from the paper in the same way as was done on the pen recorders. An electrocardiograph is normally standardised to inscribe 1 mm for 0.1 mV (100 µV) of potential deviation. The thin horizontal lines are also 1 mm apart, representing 0.1 mV and two thick lines are 5 mm apart, representing 0.5 mV. It is very important to keep the calibrations of both time and amplitude recorded on every ECG.

ECG lead system

Body surface ECGs are routinely recorded with 12 leads from the defined positions. ECG leads, particularly the chest ones should be accurately placed. The ECG lead system consists of bipolar and unipolar leads, the former recording the potential difference between any two given electrodes and the latter the potential from the sites where the electrodes are located with respect to a derived reference potential.

The three bipolar limb leads, I, II and III are connected as (figure 4-2):

Lead I: positive electrode to the left arm and negative to the right arm,

Lead II: positive electrode to the left leg and negative to the right arm,

Lead III: positive electrode to the left leg and negative to the left arm.

Therefore, the ECGs recorded by the three standard leads are the potential differences between the signals measured at the left arm (L), right arm (R) or left leg (F).

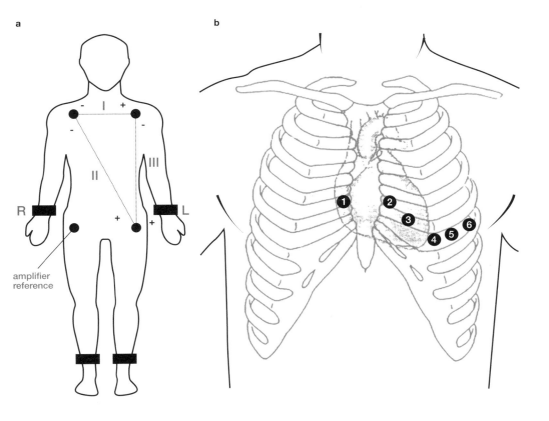

Figure 4-2 Illustrations of ECG lead placement (a) shows limb leads and (b) shows chest leads

The three augmented unipolar limb leads, avR, avL and avF, are connected to the right arm, left arm and left leg, respectively, by the same electrodes as the bipolar leads. They are recording the potential difference between a signal measured at a given limb and the average of the other two.

The unipolar chest leads (or precordial leads) are designed to record the potential difference between the given chest electrode and the average of the three limbs. The average potential of the three limbs is theoretically zero, and was originally considered as central terminal or zero potential reference point. The chest leads are arranged as:

V1: fourth intercostal space at the right sternal border,

V2: fourth intercostal space at the left sternal border,

V3: equidistant between V2 and V4,

V4: fifth intercostal space in the left midclavicular line, all the remaining chest electrodes are placed at the same horizontal plane as V4,

V5: anterior axillary line,

V6: midaxillary line.

Preparations

As with any other biological recording, the art of acquiring a good ECG consists of obtaining the optimal signal to noise ratio. The basic ECG signal is of low voltage and cannot be increased. It is thus essential to reduce the noise which is amplified along with the signal to degrade the final trace. Sources of noise include the mains alternating current, which should have been removed by a differential amplifier in the ECG recorder, poor skin contact of the electrodes, patient muscle tremor and other electrical signals. Thus every effort should be made to reduce noise interference.

The procedure should be briefly explained to the patient and its safety reassured. This may reduce patients' anxiety which can cause muscular motion, thus artifacts. In patients with uncontrollable muscular tremor, the electrodes of the limb leads can be placed in the proximal portion of the extremities. By doing so, the interference from muscular tremor will be reduced without affecting ECG signal transmission.

The couch should be big and stable enough to support the whole body of the patient and enable them to be completely relaxed. The electrodes should be placed in well exposed sites and thus shaving is, sometimes, necessary. Using pasted adhesive electrodes is helpful to obtain good contact between the electrodes and skin to eliminate spurious interference. Alcohol or acetone pads should not be used as they impair the electrode contact with the skin.

One or more filters are normally incorporated in an electrocardiograph, aiming to reduce the influence of muscular tremor or other artifacts on the ECG and so improve its aesthetic appearance. Filters should be used with great caution as they compromise the fidelity of the ECG signals. So for a diagnostic ECG, filters are only used as a last resort and the fact that they have been used should be recorded.

Safety considerations

Modern electrocardiographs are required to meet appropriate safety standards in order to minimise the risk of electric shock. The pre-amplifier circuits connecting the ECG cables and electrodes are isolated from the main power supply circuits and main power earth. This indicates that, should the patient be connected to any other equipment using mains referenced voltages, no current will flow to them.

The safety standards also require ECG recorders to restrict current leakage to safe levels in the event of faulty conditions, such as the mains plug being wired incorrectly or the patient touching some other equipment that is faulty.

QUESTIONS & ANSWERS

1 Are there any non-cardiac conditions affecting ECG recording?

A Yes. A lot of non-cardiac conditions may affect the ECG. For instance, the amplitude of the QRS complex (and all the other waveforms) is reduced where there is obesity, emphysema and peripheral oedema regardless of aetiology; electrolyte disturbances can distort ECG waveforms (particularly T wave) and cause cardiac arrhythmias; and anti-psychotic drugs can cause QT prolongation.

2 What are the pros and cons of an ECG machine which provides a single lead ECG?

A If the machine can produce a full body surface ECG lead by lead, you may use the ECG in the same way as you do a simultaneously recorded 12-lead ECG. Such ECG machines, usually slightly aged, may not provide any measurements or interpretation. It is therefore very important for the users to have basic ECG knowledge.

Some single lead ECG machines are designed to monitor heart rhythm. They should not be used for diagnostic ECGs.

05 INDICATIONS FOR ELECTROCARDIOGRAPHY

Electrocardiography, with over a century-long history in clinical practice, has much to offer community medicine. It is probably the most commonly used clinical tool certainly in both cardiology and general medicine. The ECG should be used in a sensible and cost-effective way as unnecessary investigations will add strain to an already over stretched health care system and cause anxiety to patients. Only patients with conditions for which an ECG is useful should have an ECG or serial ECGs.

LEARNING POINTS

1 The ECG is the most commonly used diagnostic tool in both primary and hospital care.

2 The ECG can be used to monitor cardiac patients or as a screening tool.

3 Exercise ECG is mainly used to diagnose coronary artery disease.

4 24-hour ECG is useful in diagnosing arrhythmias.

Patients with known cardiovascular disease or heart failure

An ECG is strongly recommended in all patients with known cardiovascular disease or heart failure during follow-up, even in the community. The frequency of follow-up ECGs depends on the clinical condition. In patients with new symptoms, serial ECGs are needed and, in stable patients, an occasional ECG will suffice. An ECG is also used to monitor therapeutic effects or side-effects of medications which are known to cause ECG changes, e.g. digoxin. Finally, all patients under this category should have an ECG before any surgery.

Patients with suspected cardiovascular disease or at high risk of cardiovascular events

All patients with suspected cardiovascular disease or at high risk of cardiovascular events should have an ECG in their first consultation at a GP's clinic. Follow-up ECGs are not routinely required. It is, nevertheless, recommended that patients under this category should have ECGs before any surgery or if they are on medication which may affect the ECG or cause arrhythmias.

Patients without known or suspected cardiovascular disease

There is no evidence that an ECG can offer useful information in patients who have not been diagnosed or suspected to have heart disease. Thus, an ECG is not recommended in patients in this category.

However, ECGs are recommended in all those over the age of 40 years who are undergoing a major operation. Similarly, ECGs should be recorded for those who are to receive medication which is known to affect the ECG or cardiac function. An ECG probably should be included in the physical examination programme, particularly for those who are in a special profession, such as a pilot, a public vehicle driver or a HGV driver.

Indications for exercise ECG and 24-hour ECG

Exercise ECG and 24-hour ECG monitoring are both useful tools even in community medicine, although they are more commonly, but not exclusively, requested by hospital doctors. Exercise ECG is the most simple and most readily available test for diagnosing coronary artery disease, and is accessible to almost all GPs. This test is indicated and probably provides clinically useful information in young patients (under 40 years) of both genders with typical anginal chest pain, those with atypical chest pain over 35 years in men and over 40 years in women, and all those over 60 years with non-anginal chest pain. As rapid access chest pain clinics become increasingly available, all the patients mentioned above are appropriate referrals for such a service.

24-hour ECG monitoring is also useful in community medicine, often serving for reassurance purposes and avoiding cardiology referrals. All patients with a complaint of unexplained syncope, near syncope or palpitations occurring a few times a week should be referred for 24-hour ECGs. But it is not helpful in patients with isolated ectopics or chronic atrial fibrillation with good ventricular rate control.

QUESTIONS & ANSWERS

1 Is the ECG a useful screening tool? Should we integrate it into our new patient check–up?

A Yes, even a resting ECG is very useful in screening. While an abnormal ECG indicates various cardiac pathologies, a normal ECG can exclude heart failure at a 70-80% confidence. It is routinely used as a part of pre-operative assessment. It may be advisable that new patients over 40 years of age have an ECG to excluded possible cardiac pathology.

2 Are there any particular patients who should not be referred for exercise ECG?

A Yes. Exercise ECG is not suitable for everybody. Contraindications for exercise ECG include systemic illness, severe hypertension, severe aortic stenosis, recent acute myocardial infarction, unstable angina and any systemic infection. There are some other conditions that prevent patients from exercising or make the interpretation difficult. This group includes arthritis, COPD, obesity, atrial fibrillation, bundle branch block pattern and existing ST-T changes.

3 What is the difference between a 24-hour ECG and a Holter monitor?

A They are the same. Dr Norman Holter invented the method of recording the ECG continuously for 24 hours, thus the 24-hour ECG is named after him. A 24-hour ECG is also known as a 24-hour ambulatory ECG monitor.

4 What is an event recorder?

A Like a 24-hour ECG, an event recorder can register ECG continuously or as activated by patients, but for a much longer time until an event (patient symptom) has occurred. The ECG is interpreted along with the reported symptom. This is particularly useful in patients whose symptoms are infrequent.

5 Why are patients with a bundle branch block pattern on resting ECG not suitable for exercise ECG?

A This is because these patients invariably have ST-T changes on the resting ECG already which make the interpretation of the exercise ECG less reliable. Similarly, in patients with left ventricular hypertrophy, there are often ST-T changes on their resting ECG, and exercise ECG is not as reliable as in those without left ventricular hypertrophy.

6 Is an exercise ECG still useful in patients with atrial fibrillation?

A It is still useful if the main concern is about symptoms. However, when the main issue is diagnosing inducible ischaemia, atrial fibrillation will make the assessment difficult because of the variable RR interval.

7 Should patients discontinue their medication before an exercise test?

A Yes, if the medication has been prescribed for treating angina. Patients are advised not to take beta blockers (some physicians advise their patients not to take nitrates as well) for at least 24 hours before the test.

06 ECG INTERPRETATION

A simple ECG can provide us with useful information and enables us to offer effective treatment. However, it needs appropriate interpretation. Despite the increasing number of ECGs recorded either in hospitals or in the community, the information they carry is probably underused. Their interpretation has gradually deteriorated over recent decades, coinciding with the development of cardiac imaging techniques.

LEARNING POINTS

1 ECG interpretation demands clinical information also.

2 Familiarity with pattern recognition is needed.

General view of the ECG

Basic patient information is needed before interpreting an ECG, including the patient's age and sex, clinical diagnosis and the indication for an ECG. Recording quality and techniques are vital in the preparation of an ECG report and therefore should be taken into consideration. These include voltage calibration (usually 0.1 mV/mm), paper speed (usually 25 mm/sec) and any filter used. Therefore, one must bear in mind that poor recording quality can be misleading and should be avoided, filters can improve the appearance of ECG traces but at the expense of fidelity.

Simple approach to ECG interpretation

ECG interpretation depends on information from all 12 leads, which sounds daunting to those whose daily routine does not include ECG interpretation. It is, however, achievable if a simple yet systematic approach is followed. Basic information including cardiac rhythm, heart rate and time measurements are normally printed out by modern ECG machines, and ECG morphology or pattern recognition becomes the cornerstone of interpretation.

ECG pattern recognition can be readily achieved by the "one-sequence-two-elements" tactic. One sequence is P, QRS and T (U), which helps avoid missing out any segment in the ECG. Two elements are amplitude (voltage) and time, the former representing the amount of activated myocardial mass and the latter reflecting the conduction speed.

The other simple way to identify ECG morphology is to detect the absence or addition of wave forms. The absence of a deflection is actually a major feature of some arrhythmias (e.g. absent P wave or QRS complex), or represents myocardial damage (e.g. the diminished T wave in ischaemia). An extra R wave of the QRS complex is a key feature of complete bundle branch block (see page 56) and a P wave with two peaks left atrial enlargement or intra-atrial conduction delay (see page 53).

Limitations of an ECG

The ECG has been the most commonly used test in clinical cardiology and it has proven to be invaluable in caring for patients with or without a definite cardiac condition. However, like any other clinical tool, the ECG should only be interpreted after an appropriate history is taken and a physical examination, and this should be interpreted ideally by the doctor who is directly responsible for the patient's care. This is extremely relevant for primary care.

The most important and probably most common ECG report is "normal ECG", but it is not the easiest diagnosis to make. Regardless of dealing with a normal ECG or an abnormal ECG, we must realise that there are limitations in electrocardiography as in any other technology.

1 The ECG may not reflect aetiology

The ECG diagnosis of left ventricular hypertrophy is made on the voltage criteria, and can be found in a normal young man as well as in patients with severe aortic stenosis or hypertension - the former is considered a physiologic hypertrophy and the latter a pathologic hypertrophy. Similarly, an abnormally tall T wave, particularly in chest leads, can occur in patients with acute myocardial infarction or in those with hyperkalaemia.

2 The ECG diagnosis may not be pathological or anatomical

First or second degree heart block does not represent any discontinuity of conduction tissue between the atrium and the ventricle. However, a pathological Q wave is the result of dead myocardium.

3 There is no simple correlation between the extent of ECG abnormalities and that of underlying disease

Patients with coronary artery disease may have a normal resting ECG. The absence of an unremarkable septal q wave indicates significant myocardial disease, while an obvious ECG pattern, complete right bundle branch block, can be a totally benign condition.

4 An abnormal ECG can be recorded in conditions other than heart disease

Electrolyte disturbances, hypothermia, hyperventilation or obesity can all cause ECG abnormalities.

5 Sometimes repeated or serial ECGs are required

In an evolving cardiac condition that is developing acutely or chronically, the ECG may be normal. It is therefore important to record follow-up ECGs to monitor the progression of the condition, for instance in acute myocardial infarction and left ventricular hypertrophy caused by high blood pressure.

07 MOST COMMON ECG ABNORMALITIES IN PRIMARY CARE

As in hospital care, the ECG is one of the most commonly used tests in general practice. Though the reason for recording ECGs varies greatly, common abnormal findings in primary care are few, mainly ST-T changes and ectopic beats.

LEARNING POINTS

1 The most common ECG abnormalities are ST changes and ectopic beats.

2 These abnormalities are found in patients as well as in normal subjects.

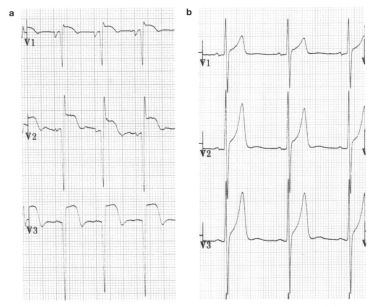

Figure 7-1 (a) ST elevation in acute myocardial infarction and (b) early repolarisation in a young (23 year old male) normal subject

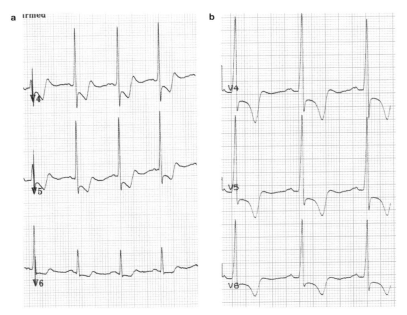

Figure 7-2 Two left chest lead ECGs recorded in (a) a patient with chest pain and subsequently confirmed to have two vessel coronary artery disease and (b) in a patient with poorly controlled hypertension and left ventricular hypertrophy on echo. This illustrates that the pattern of ST depression is not helpful in differentiating the two underlying conditions

ST-T changes

A normal ST segment is a horizontal (isoelectric) line between the end of the QRS complex and the onset of the T wave. It signifies that the heart is fully depolarised and no current flow is registered. The deviation from the baseline, either upward (ST elevation) or downward (ST depression), is defined as abnormal ST.

ST elevation

The most common and significant reason for ST elevation is acute myocardial infarction (figure 7-1a) although an increasing number of patients with acute myocardial infarction do not present with ST elevation (*Heart* 2005;**91**:1141). ST elevation can occur in acute pericarditis (see page 93: t wave alternan). Finally, ST elevation may be a normal variation particularly in young males of African origin. Such ST elevation, usually in chest leads, is referred to as early repolarisation (figure 7-1b).

ST depression

ST depression can be the result of many causes, such as myocardial ischaemia, left ventricular hypertrophy, cardiomyopathy, drug effect (e.g. digoxin) and hyperventilation. Though there are different patterns of ST depression, it is not advisable to make a pathological diagnosis based on the ST depression pattern (figure 7-2).

Ectopic beats

Ectopic beats, or premature cardiac beats, usually result from increased spontaneous firing of the conduction system below the sinus node. They usually occur before the normally conducted beats and are thus referred to as premature beats, pre-systole or extra-systole. They are very common even in structurally normal hearts and classified according to their origin (focus): atrial, junctional and ventricular ectopics (figures 7-3 to 7-9). Frequent ectopics may form bigeminy when they occur after every normal beat or trigeminy when one ectopic follows two normal beats, or couplets when ectopics come in twos. Sometimes the ventricular ectopic beats are generated from more than one focus and they are then referred to as multifocal ventricular ectopics. Strictly speaking, ectopics are not arrhythmias unless there are more than three consecutive ectopic beats which is defined as tachycardia, hence arrhythmia.

Asymptomatic ectopic beats carry no clinical significance. However, frequent ventricular ectopics which do not diminish with exertion may indicate myocardial ischaemia particularly in those with a high probability of the diagnosis.

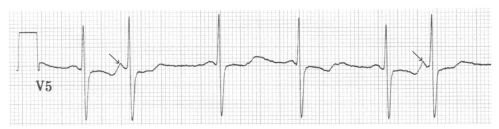

Figure 7-3 This ECG shows atrial ectopics (arrow), the ectopic P wave and sinus P waves are pointing to the same direction suggesting the ectopic focus is in the right atrium

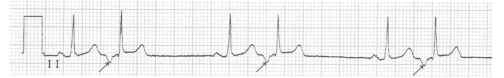

Figure 7-4 This ECG shows atrial ectopics (arrow). Note the ectopic P wave points to the opposite direction to that of the sinus P wave indicating the ectopic focus is in the left atrium, and the ectopics occur after every sinus beat thus bigeminy

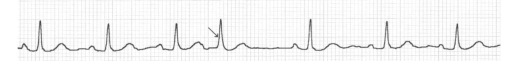

Figure 7-5 This ECG shows junction ectopic: an early but normal sized QRS complex (arrow) without a preceding P wave

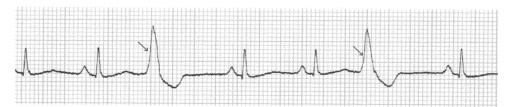

Figure 7-6 This ECG shows ventricular ectopics (arrow): early and broad QRS complexes with preceding P waves

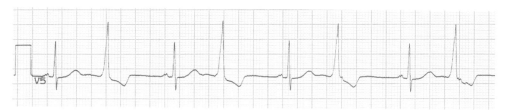

Figure 7-7 This is a typical example of ventricular ectopics, bigeminy i.e. a ventricular ectopic in every other beat

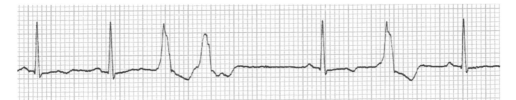

Figure 7-8 This ECG shows two consecutive ventricular ectopic beats which are referred to as a couplet. They are more likely to develop into ventricular tachycardia than those in isolation

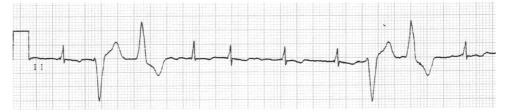

Figure 7-9 This ECG shows couplets of ventricular ectopics but the morphology is very different between the two consecutive ectopic beats, the first is downwards and second upright. They are multifocal ventricular ectopics, i.e. they are generated from different foci or areas of the heart, and are more likely to be associated with myocardial disease than isolated ventricular ectopics

QUESTIONS & ANSWERS

1 If a patient complains of palpitations and has frequent atrial ectopics, is this of clinical significance?

A It is often said that atrial ectopics are clinically insignificant if the frequency is less than 5 per minute. However, if the patient is symptomatic, even atrial ectopics should be taken seriously. Further investigations should be performed including thyroid function, 24-hour ECG and exercise ECG if the patient is over 40 years. In some other cases, an echocardiogram may also be needed to assess the cardiac morphology.

2 What are the general recommendations for managing ectopic heart beats in primary care?

A The majority of patients with ectopic heart beats have no cardiac disease and would therefore need some understanding of the ectopics, reassurance and lifestyle advice, particularly reduction of coffee and alcohol consumption. However, ectopic heart beats could be a sign of underlying cardiac disease. It is, therefore, important to take a tailored approach to managing different individuals. In the younger population, every effort should be made to exclude mitral prolapse, and in the middle-aged and the elderly population, to exclude ischaemia.

PART 2
PRACTICAL
ELECTROCARDIOGRAPHY

08 NORMAL ECG AND VARIATIONS

In daily practice, the diagnosis of a normal ECG is very important as the majority of ECGs recorded in cardiology departments are normal. Though a normal ECG does not exclude coronary artery disease, it indicates preserved ventricular function and insignificant myocardial damage, if any.

ECG morphology can be significantly different in young children compared to an adult pattern. It is very useful to recognise some normal variations which would otherwise cause unnecessary concerns. A normal ECG can be presented as abnormal due to recording errors. This chapter presents all the above mentioned ECG patterns.

LEARNING POINTS

---

1   A normal ECG is important but not always easy to confirm.

2   There are variations in 'normality'.

3   Technical errors e.g. incorrect lead placement may make an ECG abnormal.

4   A normal ECG cannot exclude cardiac pathology, but an abnormal ECG always indicates some underlying heart disease.

5   ECGs in children are different from adults.

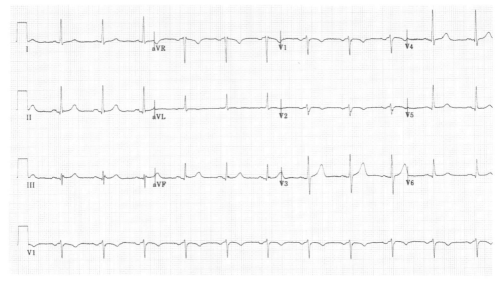

Figure 8-1 A normal ECG

Normal ECG

Case history

A 59-year-old woman with atypical chest pain was referred for electrocardiography. She did not have breathlessness or restriction on exertion. There were no abnormalities found on examination.

ECG findings

This shows sinus rhythm with a heart rate of 70 bpm. Every P wave is followed by a QRS complex. PR interval, QRS duration, QT interval and QRS axis are all normal. The morphology is normal in both the P wave and QRS complex. There is no ST shift from the isoelectric line.

ECG diagnosis: normal.

ECG diagnostic criteria. A normal ECG should meet the following criteria:

Sinus rhythm: the electric wave forms generated in the sinus node and the P wave are upright in leads II, V5 and V6, negative in avR and biphasic in V1. Every P wave is followed by a QRS complex and T wave.

Normal heart rate: 60-100 (or 55-95) bpm.

Normal PR interval: 120 – 200 ms.

Normal QRS duration: <110 ms.

Normal QRS axis: 0-90 degrees.

Normal QT interval varies with heart rate.

Normal morphology of all waveforms.

Comments

'Normal ECG' is probably the most common diagnosis in practice but not the easiest one to make. Apart from the nomenclatures described above, there are a few variations, such as sinus arrhythmia and early repolarisation. In addition, ECGs recorded in normal infants and young children appear to be abnormal if judged by adult ECG criteria, and misplacement of the electrodes can make a normal ECG abnormal. All these are illustrated in the following few pages.

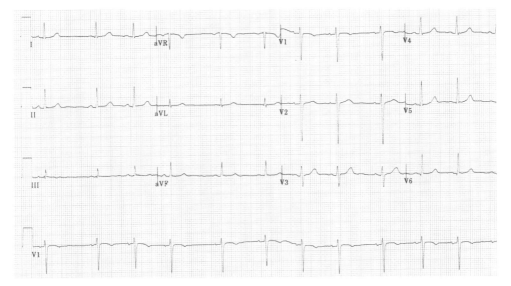

Figure 8-2 An ECG example of sinus arrhythmia

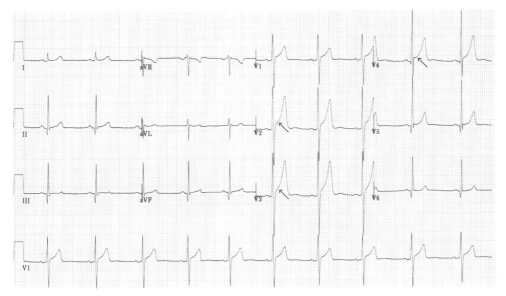

Figure 8-3 An ECG example of early repolarisation (arrows)

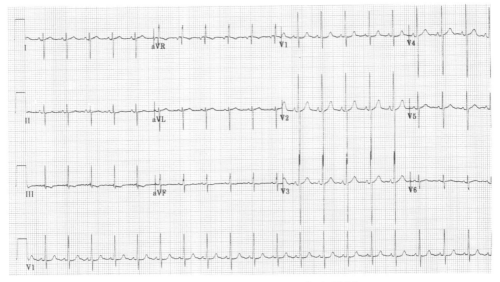

Figure 8-4 An ECG recorded in a one-month-old boy showing all paediatric ECG features

Sinus arrhythmia

This is defined as when the difference between the longest PP and shortest PP intervals exceeds 120 ms (3 mm). The ECG pictured in figure 8-2 was recorded in a 23-year-old woman.

Early repolarisation

This is ST elevation in the absence of cardiac pathology, often associated with tall T waves and QRS complexes. This ECG was recorded in a 40-year-old man who complained of atypical chest pain with a normal echocardiogram and a normal exercise ECG (figure 8-3).

Paediatric ECG

This ECG was recorded in a one-month-old baby boy. Its main features are fast heart rate, right axis deviation, prominent R wave in the right chest leads and ST-T changes (figure 8-4). They are all normal findings in this age group but highly abnormal if found in adults. Paediatric ECG features usually turn to an adult's pattern between the age of 6 and 10 years.

ECG electrode misplacement

The most common mistake is limb lead reversal, i.e. left arm lead placed on the right arm and vice versa. This mimics dextrocardia. The first ECG (figure 8-5a) was recorded with the limb leads reversed and the second (figure 8-5b) was recorded with ECG leads in the correct position (note the dramatic changes in all limb leads).

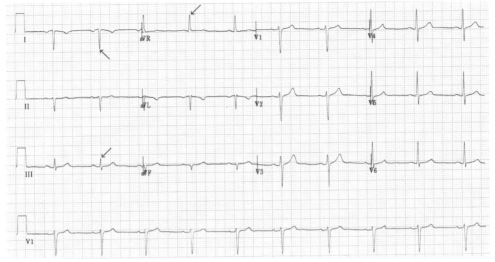

a

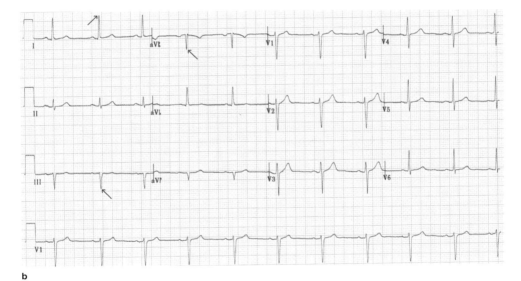

b

Figure 8-5 ECGs recorded in a normal subject with (a) misplaced and (b) normal ECG leads

09 SINUS BRADYCARDIA

LEARNING POINTS

1 Sinus rhythm with a heart rate below 60 bpm is called sinus bradycardia.

2 It is very common in normal healthy subjects, it is also common in patients on any medication which slows down heart rate, particularly beta blockers.

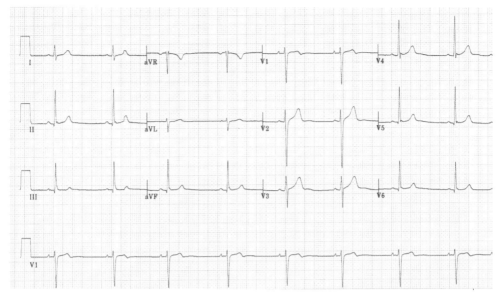

Figure 9-1 An ECG example of sinus bradycardia

Sinus bradycardia

Case history

This ECG (figure 9.1) was recorded in a 57-year-old man, who was found to have a slow pulse rate but reported no symptoms. Physical examination was normal.

ECG findings

This shows sinus rhythm - every P wave is followed by a QRS complex. The heart rate is 50 bpm and PR interval, QRS duration, QT interval and QRS axis are all normal. The morphology of the ECG is normal as well.

ECG diagnosis: sinus bradycardia.

ECG diagnostic criteria for sinus bradycardia: a heart rate below 60 bpm is defined as bradycardia and, if in sinus rhythm, as sinus bradycardia.

Comments

Sinus bradycardia is a common finding in both normal subjects and in cardiac patients who either have conduction disturbances or are on cardiac medication (including beta blockers, some calcium channel blockers, digoxin and amiodarone).

Sinus bradycardia in normal subjects or in asymptomatic patients requires no further action.

What to do next

It is important to exclude cardiac causes for bradycardia even in asymptomatic patients. Exercise ECG can clarify the chronotropic response (heart rate changes) and 24-hour ECG can exclude long sinus pauses. In symptomatic (syncope and dizziness) patients who may suffer from sick sinus syndrome, a permanent pacemaker is strongly indicated (see page 56).

10 SINUS TACHYCARDIA

LEARNING POINTS

1 Sinus rhythm with a heart rate over 100 bpm is called sinus tachycardia.

2 It can be found in both normal subjects and patients with cardiac or non-cardiac conditions.

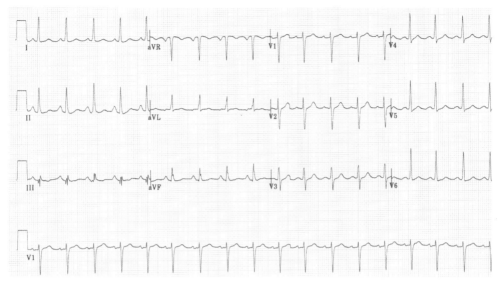

Figure 10-1 An ECG example of sinus tachycardia

Sinus tachycardia

Case history

This ECG (figure 10.1) was recorded in a 75-year-old woman waiting for a gynaecological operation. She had no cardiac symptoms except for some anxiety.

ECG findings

This shows sinus rhythm - every P wave is followed by a QRS complex. The heart rate is 110 bpm and PR interval, QRS duration, QT interval and QRS axis are all normal. The morphology of the ECG is normal as well.

ECG diagnosis: sinus tachycardia.

ECG diagnostic criteria for sinus tachycardia: a heart rate over 100 bpm and in sinus rhythm is defined as sinus tachycardia.

Comments

Sinus tachycardia is a common finding in both normal subjects and in patients with or without a cardiac condition. Anxiety, emotion, exertion, temperature, hyperthyroidism, anaemia and infection are the common non-cardiac causes for sinus tachycardia. Sinus tachycardia is also associated with heart failure and angina.

Sinus tachycardia in normal subjects or in asymptomatic patients requires no further action. However, appropriate investigations should be carried out, particularly in those with persistent sinus tachycardia.

What to do next

It is important to find the underlying cause for sinus tachycardia even in asymptomatic patients. Minimum investigation includes full blood count, thyroid function, echocardiography and exercise ECG, as appropriate.

11 ATRIOVENTRICULAR CONDUCTION ABNORMALITIES

When the cardiac conduction system is affected by any pathology, the body surface ECG is the most commonly used and yet reliable tool for detection. The common conduction abnormalities include impaired conduction in the atrioventricular junction (heart block) and bundle of His or its branches (bundle branch block).

LEARNING POINTS

1 Heart block or atrioventricular (AV) block includes a variety of conduction disturbances, ranging from the benign first degree heart block (prolonged PR interval) to complete heart block requiring a pacemaker.

2 Advanced heart block is often associated with underlying heart disease.

3 Serial ECGs or imaging tests may be necessary in monitoring patients with AV block.

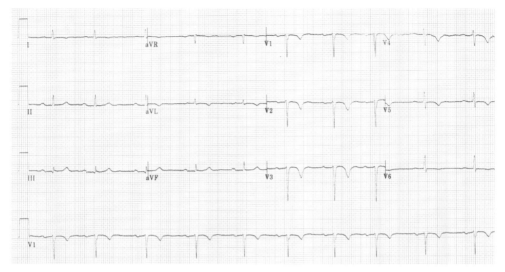

Figure 11-1 An ECG example of first degree heart block

First degree heart block

Case history

A 76-year-old man who had undergone a coronary bypass operation for three-vessel coronary artery disease is currently asymptomatic.

ECG findings

This shows sinus rhythm with a heart rate 60 bpm (figure 11-1). Every P wave is followed by a QRS complex. The PR interval is 220 ms, but QRS duration, QT interval and QRS axis are all normal. The T wave is inverted in all chest leads, I and avL.

ECG diagnosis: first degree heart block and T wave inversion.

ECG diagnostic criteria for first degree heart block: PR interval is prolonged over 200 ms (4 small squares).

Comments

The PR interval on this ECG is 220 ms. The T wave inversion in this case possibly indicates chronic ischaemia.

First degree heart block is a benign condition and does not need specific treatment. However, it can be a sign of endocarditis affecting the aortic root or valve. It is common in rheumatic fever which is a rare occurrence in developed countries.

Sometimes the PR interval is extremely long indicating intra-atrial conduction delay in addition to first degree heart block (figure 11-2).

What to do next

This patient should carry on with risk factor management. In future follow-up clinics, the patient should have the ECG recorded to document the progression of first degree heart block.

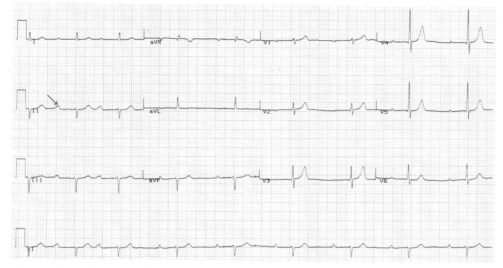

Figure 11-2 An ECG example of first degree heart block and intra-atrial conduction delay

First degree heart block and intra-atrial conduction delay

This ECG was recorded in a 90-year-old man and shows a PR interval over 370 ms and a bifid P wave i.e. two peaks, indicating left atrial enlargement or intra-atrial conduction delay. This is an example of the combination of first degree heart block and intra-atrial conduction delay probably secondary to atrial dilatation (figure 11-2).

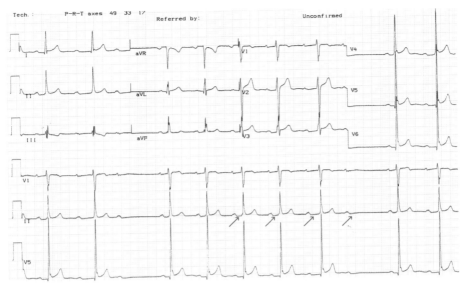

Figure 11-3 An ECG example of Mobitz type I second degree heart block

Second degree heart block

Mobitz type I (Wenckebach) block

Case history

A 32-year-old man presented with occasional "missing heart beats" but was otherwise healthy.

ECG findings

This shows sinus rhythm with a heart rate below 60 bpm (figure 11-3). Occasionally there is no QRS complex following a P wave. The PR interval progressively increases from 200 to 350 ms (arrows), but QRS duration, QT interval and QRS axis are all normal. The QRS amplitude is high indicating left ventricular hypertrophy (page 78).

ECG diagnosis: Mobitz type I (Wenckebach) second degree heart block and left ventricular hypertrophy

ECG diagnostic criteria for second degree Mobitz type I heart block: progressive prolongation of the PR interval until the P wave fails conducting to the ventricle, resulting in a QRS complex drop-out.

Comments

This ECG shows gradual prolongation of the PR interval from 200 ms to 350 ms. Sometimes, there is no QRS complex following the P wave (see cardiac beat before the first arrow).

The sum of SV2 and RV6 is well over 4.0 mV (40 mm) indicating left ventricular hypertrophy.

Mobitz type I second degree heart block is commonly found in patients with myocardial disease, such as cardiomyopathy, coronary artery disease and myocarditis. Occasionally it can be found in apparently healthy subjects.

What to do next

This patient should be referred for an echocardiogram to establish whether there is myocardial disease and a 24-hour ECG to identify more advanced heart block.

Mobitz type I heart block does not require pacing in addition to the treatment for the underlying pathology. Pacemaker insertion is indicated if it develops into more advanced heart block or the patient becomes symptomatic with syncope or dizziness.

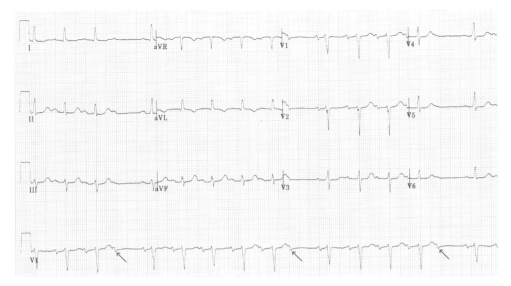

Figure 11-4 An ECG example of Mobitz type II second degree heart block

Mobitz type II block

Case history

A 59-year-old man presented with exertional breathlessness. He is a smoker and has been treated for hypertension.

ECG findings

This shows sinus rhythm with a heart rate below 80 bpm (figure 11-4). The PR interval is just over 200 ms. Some P waves are not followed by a QRS complex i.e. QRS drop-out (arrows). QRS duration, QT interval and QRS axis are all normal.

ECG diagnosis: Mobitz type II second degree heart block.

ECG diagnostic criteria for second degree Mobitz type II heart block: occasional QRS drop-out is the key feature of Mobitz type II heart block, but the relation between the P wave and QRS complex is constant in all the other cardiac cycles. The PR interval can be normal or prolonged.

Comments

This ECG shows a QRS drop-out in every four to six cardiac cycles and a long but constant PR interval.

This is a more advanced heart block than the Mobitz type I. Similarly, it is commonly found in patients with myocardial disease, such as cardiomyopathy, coronary artery disease and myocarditis. It requires further investigation into the aetiology and preparation for pacemaker implantation.

What to do next

This patient should be referred to cardiology for further investigation and management. Investigations include exercise ECG or angiography for coronary artery disease, echocardiography for myocardial disease and a 24-hour ECG for symptomatic complete heart block or arrhythmias.

Mobitz type II heart block requires pacing in most cases except in acute myocardial infarction where full recovery is very likely.

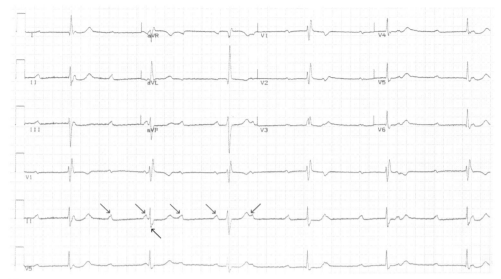

Figure 11-5 An ECG example of third degree (complete) heart block

Third degree (complete) heart block

Case history

A 67-year-old woman, who had been healthy and complained of fatigue recently, was found to have slow heart rates of 40 to 50 bpm on examination.

ECG findings

This shows sinus rhythm and there are more P waves (blue arrows) than QRS complexes (black arrow) as P waves are not followed by QRS complexes (figure 11-5). The atrial (P) rate is 75 bpm and ventricular (QRS) rate is 35 to 40 bpm. Both QRS duration and QT interval are slightly prolonged though the QRS axis is within normal limits. The QRS complex shows an rSR in V1, V2 and V3.

ECG diagnosis: complete heart block with right bundle branch block QRS pattern.

ECG diagnostic criteria for complete heart block:
sinus P waves with a normal atrial rate (60 -100 bpm) are not followed by a QRS complex, showing no relation between the two. The ventricular rate is slower than the atrial rate.

Comments

This ECG meets the criteria for complete heart block or third degree atrioventricular block. Most patients with complete heart block die within weeks of the diagnosis if untreated. As the ventricular rate was very slow, the patient was referred urgently for pacemaker implantation although there was no history of blackout or fainting (Stokes-Adams attack).

Various cardiac pathologies can cause complete heart block, e.g. coronary artery disease, cardiomyopathy and aortic valve disease.

Complete heart block may occur in children and is classified as congenital complete heart block where the QRS duration is usually within normal limits. However, many acquired complete heart block patients have a totally normal QRS duration.

What to do next

All patients with complete heart block should be referred to cardiology for pacemaker implantation. Further investigations are often needed, such as 24-hour ECG, echocardiography and coronary angiography. Symptomatic patients should have pacemaker insertion without delay.

12 BUNDLE BRANCH BLOCK

Unlike atrioventricular block discussed earlier, bundle branch block occurs at the ventricular level, i.e. in the bundle of His and its branches or sub-branches or fascicles. It is calcified according to where the delayed conduction occurs. There are combinations of different types of conduction delay, named as bifascicular or trifascicular blocks.

LEARNING POINTS

1   Conduction abnormalities at the ventricular level are called bundle branch block or fascicular block.

2   Both QRS duration and morphology are used to classify the types of bundle branch block.

3   Right bundle branch block is considered to be benign; left bundle branch block and bifascicular or trifascicular block may indicate underlying cardiac disease.

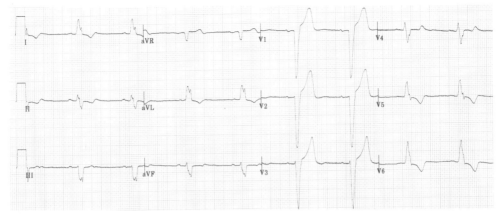

Figure 12-1 An ECG example of left bundle branch block

Left bundle branch block

Case history

An 80-year-old man with a long history of hypertension developed dyspnoea recently. There are no typical signs of congestive cardiac failure on examination.

ECG findings

This shows sinus rhythm with a slow heart rate at 52 bpm. The PR interval is normal, but QRS duration (150 ms) and QT interval (480 ms) are greatly increased. The QRS axis is leftward. The QRS complexes are M shaped in the left-sided leads, I, avL and to a lesser degree V5 and V6, where there is no septal q wave. There are global ST-T abnormalities (figure 12-1).

ECG diagnosis: sinus bradycardia, complete left bundle branch block (LBBB).

ECG diagnostic criteria for LBBB: prolonged QRS duration over 120 ms (three small squares).

Absence of septal q wave.

Dominant R wave or M shaped QRS complex in left-sided leads (V5, V6, I and avL) and dominant S wave in right-sided leads.

Other ECG changes associated with LBBB include left axis deviation, increased QRS amplitude and ST-T abnormalities.

Comments

This ECG has all major features of LBBB, increased QRS duration, absence of septal q wave and M shaped QRS complexes in left-sided leads. It also shows left axis deviation and ST-T changes.

LBBB is mostly found in patients with heart disease secondary to various underlying aetiology including hypertension, coronary artery disease, aortic valve disease and cardiomyopathy. Occasionally, it can be found in a structurally normal heart based on the currently available imaging techniques.

What to do next

Apart from treating the underlying cause, further investigations are indicated particularly echocardiography which may provide information on left ventricular size and function, as well as valvular assessment. In cases with a high risk of coronary artery disease, a diagnostic angiogram should be performed.

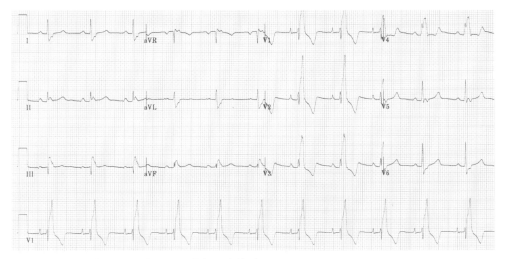

Figure 12-2 An ECG example of right bundle branch block

Right bundle branch block

Case history

A 42-year-old man with newly diagnosed hypertension came for a consultation. He was asymptomatic. Physical examination was normal.

ECG findings

This shows sinus rhythm with a heart rate at 65 bpm. The PR interval is normal, but QRS duration (180 ms) and QT interval (QTc=480 ms) are greatly increased. The QRS axis is normal to rightward. The QRS complexes are M shaped in the right-sided leads, V1 and V2. There are ST-T abnormalities, particularly in V1 and V2 (figure 12-2).

ECG diagnosis: complete right bundle branch block (RBBB).

ECG diagnostic criteria for RBBB:

Prolonged QRS duration over 120 ms.

Dominant R wave or M shaped QRS complex in right-sided leads and broadened or dominant S wave in left-sided leads.

Other ECG changes in RBBB include right axis deviation, increased QRS amplitude and ST-T abnormalities.

Comments

This ECG has all the major features of RBBB: increased QRS duration, M shaped QRS complexes in right-sided leads and ST-T changes.

RBBB is mostly found in patients with congenital heart diseases involving the right heart (e.g. atrial septal defect), hypertension, pulmonary hypertension. It can be found in structurally normal hearts. The combination of complete RBBB and left axis deviation is referred to as bifascicular block which is usually associated with myocardial disease (figure 12-5). When there is an additional long PR interval, this is trifascicular block (figure 12-6) which is a possible indication for a permanent pacemaker.

What to do next

In addition to treating the underlying cause, echocardiography should be performed to exclude any structural abnormalities.

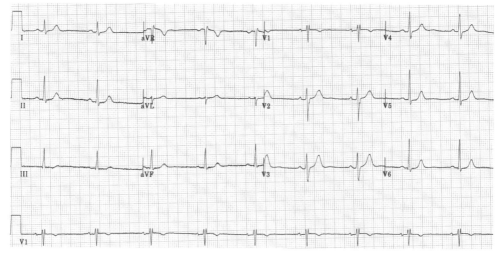

Figure 12-3 An ECG example of incomplete right bundle branch block

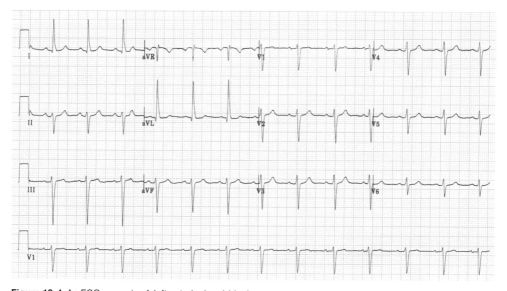

Figure 12-4 An ECG example of left anterior hemi-block

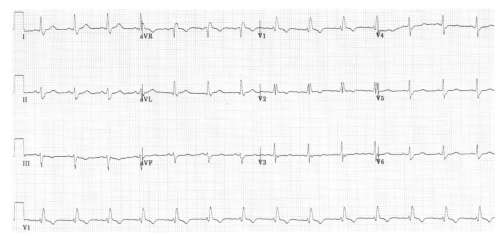

Figure 12-5 An ECG example of bifascicular block of right bundle branch block with left axis deviation

Fascicular block

Apart from complete left and right bundle branch block, there are other types of intraventricular conduction delay including incomplete left bundle branch block, incomplete right branch block, left anterior hemi-block, bifascicular block, trifascicular block and, less commonly, left posterior hemi-block.

Incomplete left/right bundle branch block

The ECG features are the same as in complete left or right bundle branch block, respectively, except the QRS duration is less than 120 ms but above 110 ms (figure 12-3). Incomplete left/right bundle branch block is less common than incomplete right bundle branch block.

Left anterior hemi-block

This is the isolated left axis deviation of the QRS complex. It is attributed to the delayed conduction in the anterior branch of the left bundle (figure 12-4).

Bifascicular block

When the abnormal conduction involves two bundles or two branches, it is referred to as bifascicular block. The most common one is complete right bundle branch block with left axis deviation suggesting conduction delay or blockage in the entire right bundle and the anterior branch of the left bundle. There is no need to treat this type of abnormal conduction rather than treating the underlying pathology (figure 12-5).

Trifascicular block

The most common type of trifascicular block is the combination of first degree heart block (a prolonged PR interval), right bundle branch block pattern and left hemi-block (left axis deviation) (figure 12-6). Symptomatic patients of this condition should have a permanent pacemaker fitted in addition to medication for possible aetiology. Asymptomatic patients need to be reviewed in cardiology regularly with a 24-hour ECG.

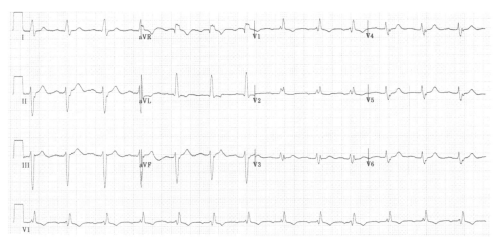

Figure 12-6 An ECG example of trifascicular block

13 ARRHYTHMIAS

When cardiac electrical activity is initiated other than in the sinus node, the cardiac rhythm is referred to as an arrhythmia which can be irregular or regular. The clinical consequences are determined by the nature of the arrhythmia.

Although any successive three or more ectopic cardiac beats are defined as an arrhythmia, ectopic beats may not be identified in some arrhythmias, for example, atrial fibrillation, atrial flutter and ventricular fibrillation. In atrial flutter, 2:1 or 3:1 conduction is used to describe the presence of one QRS complex for every two or three flutter waves.

LEARNING POINTS

1   The most common arrhythmia is atrial fibrillation.

2   Atrial fibrillation and flutter are special cases of supraventricular arrhythmia (SVT), associated with increased risk of stroke and patients should be anticoagulated.

3   SVT could be the only manifestation of an accessory pathway and often occurs in a structurally normal heart.

4   Both ventricular tachycardia (VT) and SVT with aberrant conduction are broad QRS complex tachycardias. When the differentiation is difficult, the patient should be treated as VT.

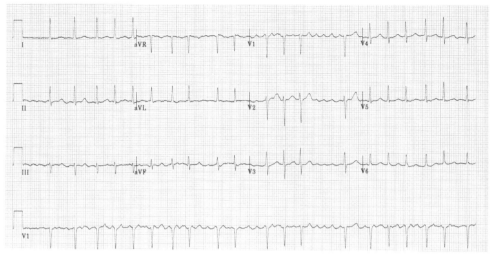

Figure 13-1 An ECG example of atrial fibrillation

Atrial fibrillation

Case history

A 68-year-old man complained of breathlessness for a few months. He had been treated for hypertension and hypothyroidism for a long time. On examination his pulses were irregular.

ECG findings

This shows no regular P waves but there are a lot of irregular waves between QRS complexes. These totally irregular deflects are called fibrillation waves. The ventricular rate (frequency of the QRS complexes) is above 100 bpm. QRS duration, QT interval and QRS axis are all normal (figure 13-1).

ECG diagnosis: atrial fibrillation.

ECG diagnostic criteria for atrial fibrillation:
Instead of regular P waves for each QRS complex, there are irregular (in both amplitude and duration) fibrillation waves between QRS complexes.

Comments

On this ECG, there are a few fibrillation waves for each QRS complex. The ventricular rate is over 100 bpm, which suggests that the arrhythmia may have caused the symptoms.

Atrial fibrillation is the most common arrhythmia and increases with age. It is often a part of a cardiac (mitral valve disease, coronary heart disease and cardiomyopathy) or a non-cardiac condition (thyroid disease, hypertension and excess alcohol consumption) (figure 13-1). It increases the risk of cardiac dysfunction, stroke and mortality. The treatment of AF includes rhythm restoration, heart rate control and anticoagulation in addition to dealing with the underlying pathology. Both medication and DC cardioversion are used to restore rhythm, bearing in mind that before DC cardioversion adequate anticoagulation is essential.

If the ventricular rate is below 85 to 90 bpm and the patient is asymptomatic, treatment may be needed for underlying pathology only (figure 13-2). On the contrary, fast atrial fibrillation (figure 13-3), even in the absence of overt heart failure, should be treated actively for rate control or rhythm restoration, preferably in hospital. This is because fast AF can lead to tachycardia-induced ventricular failure. Echocardiography is very important in providing information on cardiac structure and function.

What to do next

This patient should be referred to cardiology for rate control, rhythm restoration, and ventricular function (echocardiography) assessment and treatment. In addition, anticoagulation should be started straight away.

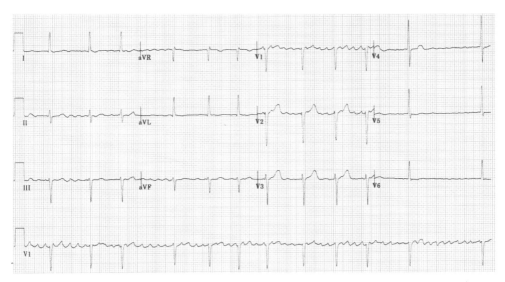

Figure 13-2 Atrial fibrillation with controlled ventricular rate recorded in a 68-year-old man who was asymptomatic

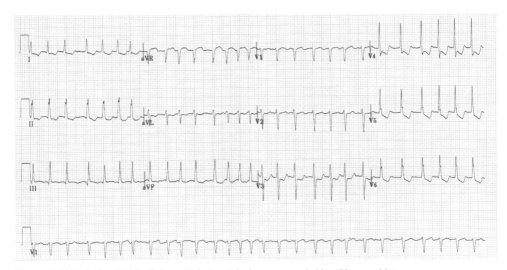

Figure 13-3 Fast AF - atrial fibrillation with fast ventricular rate recorded in a 63-year-old man

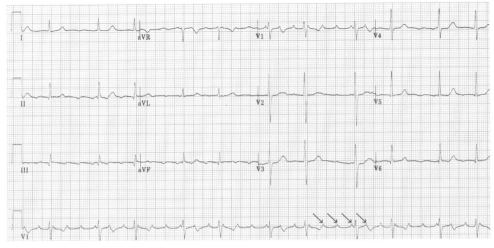

Figure 13-4 An ECG example of atrial flutter with a flutter rate of 200 bpm

Atrial flutter

Case history

An 80-year-old man treated for hypertension for a long time was found to have irregular heart beats.

ECG findings

This shows no regular P waves and, instead, there are a few small and regular waves between QRS complexes. These small waves, or flutter waves, are negative in II and positive in V1 with a rate of 200 bpm. There are far more flutter waves than QRS complexes. QRS duration, QT interval and QRS axis are all normal (figure 13-4).

ECG diagnosis: atrial flutter.

ECG diagnostic criteria for atrial flutter:

there are no P waves but flutter waves between QRS complexes. The flutter waves are of saw toothed appearance with a typical rate of 250 to 300 bpm.

Comments

On this ECG, there is one QRS complex for every two to four flutter waves (arrows), indicating a 2:1, 3:1 and 4:1 atrioventricular conduction pattern. This explains his irregular heart beats or pulse. The flutter rate here is 200 bpm, slower than that in typical atrial flutter (figure 13-5). Sometimes, atrial flutter with 2 to 1 conduction can easily be taken as sinus tachycardia if no efficient attention is paid to the "P wave" morphology (figure 13-6).

Atiral flutter is a sign of heart disease. It should be converted back to sinus rhythm by means of DC cardioversion.

What to do next

Apart from treating the existing hypertension, this patient should be referred to cardiology for cardioversion. Prior to that, however, the patient should be anticoagulated and have an echocardiogram to assess cardiac structure and function.

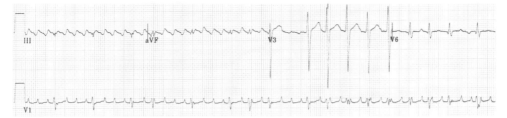

Figure 13-5 Typical atrial flutter recorded in a 54-year-old man showing variable atrioventricular conduction (flutter rate is 280 bpm and ventricular rate is about 90 bpm)

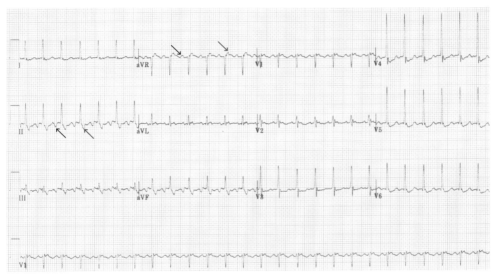

Figure 13-6 This ECG was recorded in an 81-year-old man showing atrial flutter with 2:1 conduction. Note: the flutter waves before the QRS complex is negative in lead II and positive in avR (opposite to sinus rhythm, black arrows) and the other flutter waves are buried in T waves (blue arrows)

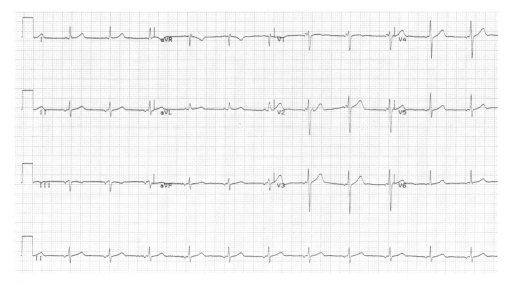

Figure 13-7 An ECG example of left atrial rhythm

Left atrial rhythm

Case history

This ECG was recorded in a 49-year-old man, who complained of newly developed fatigue. He was not on any regular medication. Physical examination was normal.

ECG findings

This shows regular rhythm with a heart rate of 70 bpm, every P wave is followed by a QRS complex, but the P wave is downward in lead II, upright in lead avR, and downward and then upright in V1, suggesting the vector direction of the P wave is the opposite to that of the sinus P wave and, hence, the impulse is generated in the left atrium. The PR interval is short but QRS duration, QT interval and QRS axis are all normal (figure 13-7).

ECG diagnosis: left atrial rhythm.

ECG diagnostic criteria for left atrial rhythm:
The key feature for left atrial rhythm is that the direction of the P wave is opposite to that of the sinus P wave.

Comments

Left atrial rhythm may occur in normal subjects and can develop into tachycardia. However, it could be a sign of coronary artery disease or other cardiac conditions. It should be distinguished from atrial fibrillation or flutter.

What to do next

Though left atrial rhythm *per se* does not need treatment, it is important to find its cause and therefore a cardiology referral is appropriate. Expected cardiac tests include exercise ECG and 24-hour ECG at least.

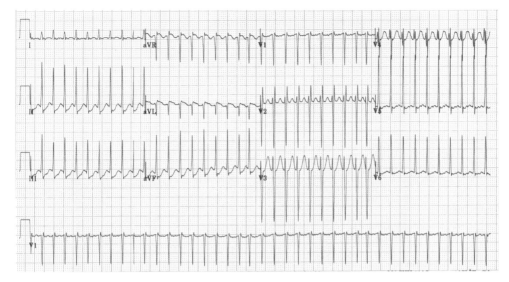

Figure 13-8 An ECG example of supraventricular tachycardia

Supraventricular tachycardia

Case history

This ECG was recorded in a 50-year-old woman, who complained of palpitations that often started suddenly. Apart from a fast pulse rate, physical examination was normal.

ECG findings

This shows that no P waves precede QRS complexes. The heart rate is over 200 bpm. QRS duration, QRS axis and QT interval are all normal (figure 13-8).

ECG diagnosis: supraventricular tachycardia (SVT).

ECG diagnostic criteria for SVT: the heart rate is at least over 150 bpm in SVT, and there is no identifiable P wave; the QRS complex is normal.

Comments

SVT usually presents as a sudden onset and sudden or gradual subsiding arrhythmia. It is most likely the result of an abnormal conduction pathway within or near the atrioventricular node causing so called "atrioventricular nodal re-entrant tachycardia (AVNRT)". The main differential diagnoses are fast atrial fibrillation and atrial flutter with 2:1 atrioventricular conduction (figure 13-9 and figure 13-10). Occasionally, there are abnormal P waves either preceding or following a QRS complex.

SVT is not commonly associated with structural heart disease other than the abnormal conduction substrate. Symptoms are directly related to the tachycardia itself. It can be terminated by Valsalva manoeuvres or carotid massage (one side at a time) (figure 13-11).

What to do next

Occasional SVT may not cause much discomfort and can be kept under observation. Recurrent or sustained SVT should be investigated and treated effectively by ablation. A routine ECG between episodes of SVT is essential to exclude other possible conduction disturbances particularly Wolff-Parkinson-White (WPW) syndrome (page 81) which commonly presents as SVT in the first instance. A subsequent important investigation is a cardiac electrophysiology study, leading to high frequency ablation therapy.

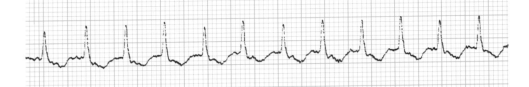

Figure 13-9 This is a SVT with a heart rate of 180 bpm. The slightly irregular QRS morphology makes it similar to fast atrial fibrillation

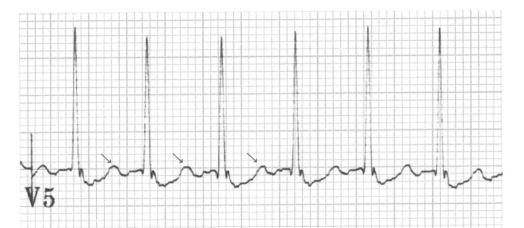

Figure 13-10 This is atrial flutter with 2:1 conduction, almost indistinguishable from SVT but for the flutter waves (arrows) which can, sometimes, be missed

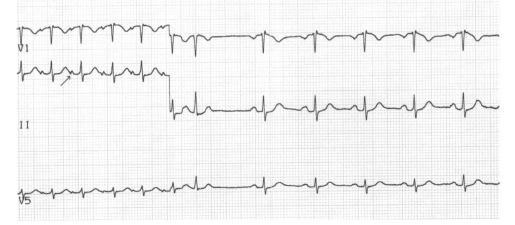

Figure 13-11 This SVT probably originated in the atrioventricular node (indicated by the abnormal P waves, arrow) and was terminated by carotid massage

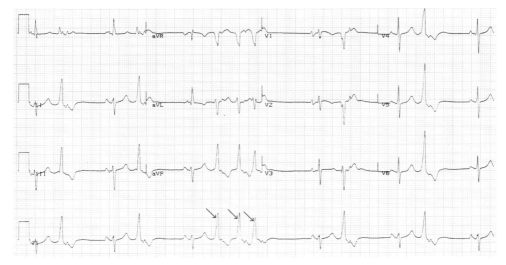

Figure 13-12 An ECG example of non-sustained ventricular tachycardia

Ventricular tachycardia (VT)

Case history

This ECG was recorded in a 79-year-old man, who complained of left-sided chest pain on exertion. He was not on any regular medication. Physical examination was normal.

ECG findings

This shows sinus rhythm with frequent ventricular ectopics, bigeminy and a run of three consecutive ventricular ectopics (arrows, figure 13-12). The heart rate is 75 bpm and some QRS complexes are preceded by P waves. In the normally conducted cardiac beats, the PR interval, QRS duration, QT interval are all normal but QRS axis shows left axis deviation (figure 13-12).

ECG diagnosis: short run of ventricular tachycardia

ECG diagnostic criteria for ventricular tachycardia: three or more consecutive ventricular ectopics are defined as ventricular tachycardia, or sustained ventricular tachycardia if lasting for more than 30 seconds.

Comments

Ventricular tachycardia occurs invariably in patients with myocardial disease particularly coronary artery disease. Sustained ventricular tachycardia can cause haemodynamic compromise and is life threatening.

Exertion-induced ventricular tachycardia is a reliable sign of significant coronary artery disease (figure 13-13).

Sometimes an ECG of SVT with aberrant conduction can be taken as ventricular tachycardia. There are various guidelines to differentiate the two. A baseline ECG or that recorded between episodes of aberrant SVT can help differentiate. However, it is advisable to treat them as ventricular tachycardia if the differentiation cannot be achieved with confidence (figure 13-14a and figure 13-14b).

What to do next

Patients with even non-sustained ventricular tachycardia warrant a cardiac referral. They should be thoroughly investigated and probably treated with appropriate antiarrhythmic agents while waiting for investigations.

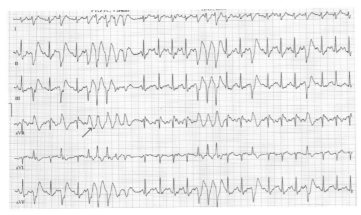

Figure 13-13 This ECG was recorded in a 65-year-old man during a treadmill exercise test. The stress-induced ventricular tachycardia (arrow) indicates inducible ischaemia

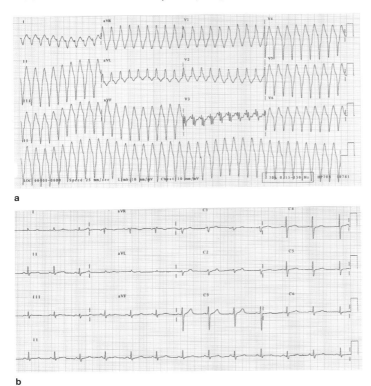

a

b

Figure 13-14 These two ECGs were recorded in a 42-year-old man who presented to A&E with palpitations. The ECG on arrival (a) shows a fast (rate of 200 bpm) broad QRS complex tachycardia, suggestive of atrial flutter 1:1 conduction (rare, rate usually over 250 bpm), ventricular tachycardia or supraventricular tachycardia with aberrant conduction. A previous ECG (b) was found to be in normal sinus rhythm with totally different QRS morphology to that in the first ECG. Thus the first ECG was ventricular tachycardia

14 CHAMBER DILATATION OR HYPERTROPHY

The dilatation or hypertrophy of any cardiac chamber can result in ECG changes. While echocardiography is a more reliable method in assessing cardiac structure, electrocardiography is more readily available than echocardiography, particularly in the community. Thus, in circumstances where echocardiography is not available, ECG can provide useful and clinically relevant information. The following ECGs and cases will illustrate how useful the ECG can be.

LEARNING POINTS

1   The duration or amplitude or both are used to diagnose chamber dilatation or hypertrophy.

2   There are often secondary changes particularly ST-T abnormalities.

3   Echocardiography is a much more reliable method than electrocardiography in assessing chamber dilatation.

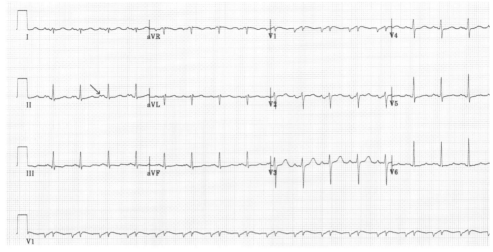

Figure 14-1 An ECG example of left atrial dilatation

Left atrial dilatation

Case history

A 56-year-old woman, who recently arrived in the UK, complained of fatigue and mild breathlessness on exertion. On auscultation, there was a soft systolic murmur in the apex but no diastolic murmur.

ECG findings

This shows sinus rhythm and every P wave is followed by a QRS complex. The heart rate is 75 bpm and PR interval, QRS duration, QT interval and QRS axis are all normal. There are two peaks (arrow) in the P waves (bifid P waves) and the P wave duration is at the upper limit of normal (figure 14-1) .

ECG diagnosis: left atrial dilatation.

ECG diagnostic criteria for left atrial dilatation: there are bifid P waves particularly in lead II, the second peak is taller than the first and the time delay between the two reaches 40 ms (1 small square) or more. There is a prominent

negative deflection of the second part of the P wave in lead V1.

Comments

This ECG shows bifid P waves in lead II and prominent negative P waves in lead V1. The time interval between the two peaks of the P wave is over 50 ms suggesting left atrial dilatation (which was confirmed by echo in this woman who suffered from mild mitral stenosis and regurgitation).

Left atrial dilatation is mainly caused by mitral valve disease, stenosis and/or regurgitation. Other cardiac pathologies including coronary artery disease, hypertension, aortic regurgitation, cardiomyopathy or chronic atrial fibrillation can also cause left atrial dilatation.

What to do next

It is very important for all patients with an ECG pattern of left atrial dilatation to have an echocardiogram, which can provide useful information on the exact atrial size and possible aetiology.

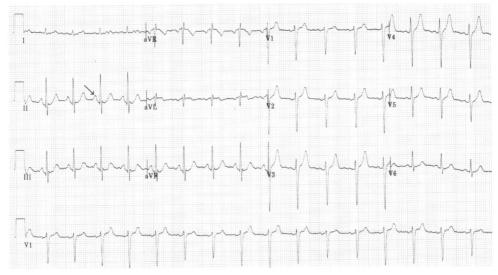

Figure 14-2 An ECG example of right atrial dilatation

Right atrial dilatation

Case history

A 58-year-old man complained of shortness of breath. No apparent abnormalities were found on physical examination.

ECG findings

This shows sinus rhythm and every P wave is followed by a QRS complex. The heart rate is approximately 100 bpm and PR interval, QRS duration, QT interval and QRS axis are all normal. The P wave is tall (arrow) in amplitude and normal in duration (figure 14-2).

ECG diagnosis: right atrial dilatation.

ECG diagnostic criteria for right atrial dilatation: high voltage (over 0.25 mV) of P waves, particularly in lead II (arrow), is the main ECG feature for right atrial dilatation.

Comments

This ECG shows an increased wave amplitude ≥ 0.25 mV in lead II.

Right atrial dilatation is mainly associated with pressure or volume overload of the right heart, particularly pulmonary hypertension and pulmonary embolism. The higher the P wave amplitude, the greater the right atrial size, though the ECG can be normal in some patients with right atrial dilatation.

When both P wave duration and amplitude are increased, it is said to be biatrial dilatation (figure 14-3).

What to do next

This patient should have an echocardiogram to assess cardiac cavity size and right ventricular systolic pressure by Doppler technique.

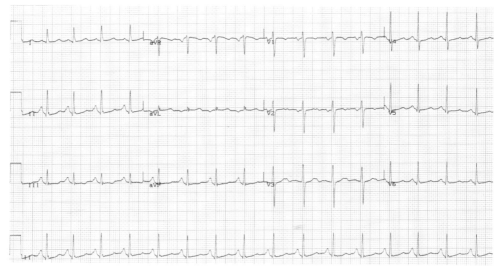

Figure 14-3 An ECG example of biatrial dilatation

Biatrial dilatation

Case history

A 49-year-old man complained of shortness of breath on minimum exertion. There was a pan systolic murmur in the apex and mild peripheral oedema on physical examination.

ECG findings

This shows sinus rhythm and every P wave is followed by a QRS complex. The heart rate is approximately 100 bpm and PR interval, QRS duration, QT interval and QRS axis are all normal. The P wave is tall in amplitude and wide in duration (figure 14-3).

ECG diagnosis: biatrial dilatation.

ECG diagnostic criteria for biatrial dilatation: the combination of a high voltage (over 0.25 mV) and prolonged duration (over 120 ms) of P waves is the main ECG diagnostic criterion.

Comments

This ECG shows an increased amplitude ≥ 0.25 mV and a prolonged duration (130 ms) of the P wave in lead II.

Biatrial dilatation is rare. It indicates heart disease with pulmonary involvement, such as dilated cardiomyopathy with secondary pulmonary hypertension and complex congenital heart disease. Sometimes, atrial dilatation on ECG does not represent dimensional enlargement but increased atrial pressure (figure 14-4).

What to do next

This patient has clinical features of heart failure and should be referred to cardiology for an echocardiogram in the first instance (this patient was confirmed echocardiographically to have dilated cardiomyopathy and biatrial dilatation). Heart failure therapy should be initiated sooner than later. Further investigation includes angiography to identify the aetiology.

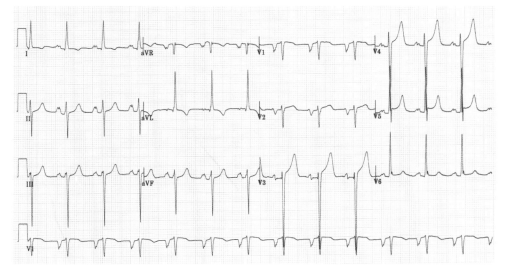

Figure 14-4 This ECG was recorded in a 37-year-old man with hypertrophic obstructive cardiomyopathy. Both atrial diameters are well within normal limits of echocardiography but the ECG shows typical biatrial dilatation

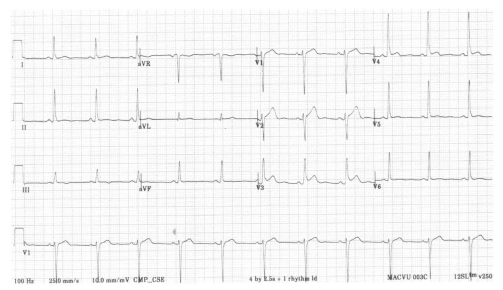

Figure 14-5 An ECG example of left ventricular hypertrophy

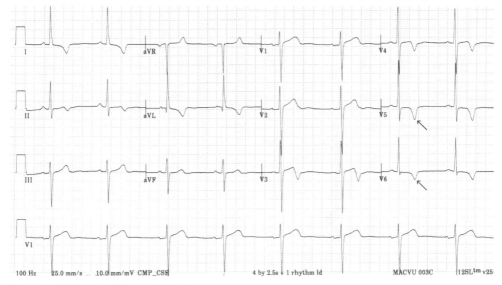

Figure 14-6 This is an ECG recorded in a 41-year-old man with hypertension indicating LVH with strain pattern (arrows)

Left ventricular hypertrophy

Case history

A 34-year-old man of African origin was recently found to have elevated blood pressure (190/112 mmHg) at a routine check-up. He is asymptomatic. Both his parents had hypertension. After 4 week's treatment including life style modification and medication, his blood pressure has been much improved (142/86 mmHg).

ECG findings

This shows sinus rhythm with a heart rate of 65 bpm. The QRS axis is normal, so are PR interval, QRS duration and QT interval. QRS amplitude is increased and indicating left ventricular hypertrophy (LVH). There is ST elevation in V1 to V5 along with flat T waves in II, III, avF and V4 to V6 (figure 14-5).

ECG diagnosis: left ventricular hypertrophy.

ECG diagnostic criteria for LVH: the ECG diagnosis of left ventricular hypertrophy is made mainly on voltage criteria:

SV1+RV5 (or RV6) ≥3.5 mV for male

SV1+RV5 (or RV6) ≥4.0 mV for female

Or avL 1.1 mV

Or SV3+ RavL ≥2.8 mV for male

SV3+ RavL ≥2.0 mV for female

Other ECG changes associated with LVH include prolongation of QRS duration, left axis deviation and ST-T changes, as seen in this case.

Comments

On this ECG, the sum of SV1 and RV5 is 4.3 mV along with ST-T changes. The ST-T changes in this case are secondary to LVH but not suggestive of myocardial ischaemia due to coronary artery disease. In more severe LVH, the ST-T changes are more profound and called "left ventricular hypertrophy with strain pattern" regardless of aetiology (figures 14-6 and 14-7).

LVH is common in hypertension and reversible with blood pressure control. Other conditions commonly causing LVH include aortic stenosis and hypertrophic cardiomyopathy. Echocardiography is more accurate than ECG in assessing the severity of LVH.

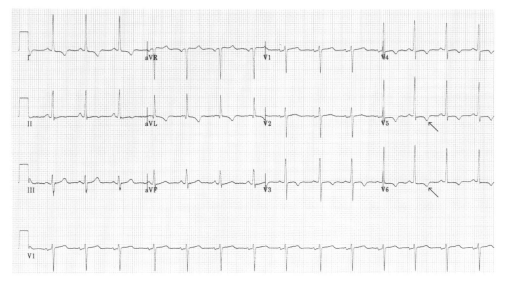

Figure 14-7 This is an ECG recorded in a 36-year-old patient with hypertrophic cardiomyopathy, again, indicating LVH with strain pattern (arrows)

What to do next

Apart from regular blood pressure monitoring, we suggest an echocardiogram to assess the severity of LVH and baseline information on left ventricular function. As LVH is an independent risk factor for cardiac events, an ECG and/or an echocardiogram probably should be repeated in a few years, in particular to assess the regression of LVH.

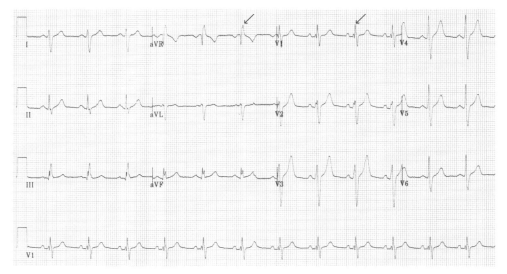

Figure 14-8 An ECG example of right ventricular hypertrophy

Right ventricular hypertrophy

Case history

A 26-year-old man was referred to cardiology because of mild dyspnoea on exertion. On auscultation, there was a 3/6 ejection systolic murmur in the pulmonary area (second intercostal space of the left sternal edge).

ECG findings

This shows sinus rhythm with a heart rate of 80 bpm. The PR interval and QT interval are both normal but the QRS duration is slightly prolonged. The QRS axis is rightward and there is prominent R wave in avR and V1. The R wave amplitude in the left chest leads (V5 and V6) is similar to that of S wave, and it is much lower in the left lateral leads (I and avL) (figure 14-8).

ECG diagnosis: right ventricular hypertrophy (RVH).

ECG diagnostic criteria for RVH: they include dominant R wave (arrows) in the right in avR or V1 and V2, and right axis deviation. The sum of R wave amplitude in V1 (or V2) and S wave in V5 or V6 is 1.1 mV or more.

Comments

The sum of R wave in V1 and S wave in V5 in this ECG is 1.4 mV and there is right axis deviation, satisfying the diagnostic criteria for right ventricular hypertrophy. As this ECG is recorded in a young patient who has an ejection systolic murmur, the most likely underlying pathology is pulmonary steonsis.

RVH commonly occurs in pulmonary disease including pulmonary stenosis, pulmonary hypertension and chronic obstructive airways disease. It can be associated with other pathologies, such as right ventricular outflow obstruction and mitral stenosis.

What to do next

This patient should have an echocardiogram to confirm or refute the diagnosis of pulmonary stenosis, and assess the severity of the lesion. It is also appropriate to refer the patient to cardiology for further management.

15 PRE-EXCITATION SYNDROME

Accessory pathway or myocardial tissue across the atrioventricular junction results in premature electrical impulse conducted from the atria to the ventricles. Such premature activity is defined as pre-excitation. The typical example of pre-excitation is Wolff-Parkinson-White syndrome.

LEARNING POINTS

1 The most common type of pre-excitation is Wolff-Parkinson-White syndrome (WPW).

2 WPW is often associated with SVT.

3 High frequency ablation offers effective treatment.

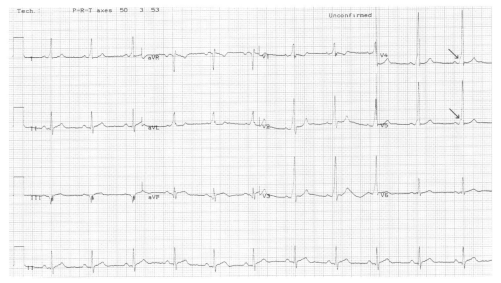

Figure 15-1 An ECG example of WPW syndrome (type A)

Wolff-Parkinson-White syndrome

Case history

This ECG (figure 15-1) was recorded in a 24-year-old man, who complained of regular palpitations which were characterised by sudden onset and offset. Physical examination was normal.

ECG findings

The ECG shows sinus P waves followed by QRS complexes, but the PR interval is short. The heart rate is 70 bpm, QRS duration is prolonged due to a slurred onset, the delta wave (arrows). Both QRS axis and QT interval are normal (figure 15-1).

ECG diagnosis: Wolff-Parkinson-White (WPW) syndrome or pre-excitation syndrome.

ECG diagnostic criteria for WPW syndrome: short PR interval, delta wave and prolonged QRS duration are the main three major features. When the main QRS deflection in V1 is positive, it is defined as type A, and when this is negative, it is defined as type B (figure 15-2), though this is a simplified classification.

Comments

There are often secondary ST-T changes. Sometimes, pre-excitation can be associated with paroxysmal SVT or atrial fibrillation.

This is an uncommon condition and associated with a structurally normal heart except for the accessory atrioventricular pathway.

What to do next

Asymptomatic WPW syndrome needs no further investigation or treatment. Patients presenting with SVT or AF should be referred to cardiology, preferably to where there are facilities for cardiac electrophysiology studies and high frequency ablation.

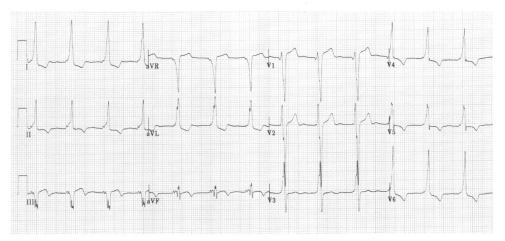

Figure 15-2 This ECG shows WPW with negative main deflection of the QRS complex in V1 and this is defined as type B WPW

16 CORONARY HEART DISEASE

LEARNING POINTS

1 An ECG is the most commonly used test for coronary artery disease.

2 An ECG help diagnose acute or chronic ischaemia, and help identify ischaemic territory.

3 Normal ECG cannot rule out coronary artery disease.

As an ECG is the direct consequence of myocardial electrical activities, myocardial disease caused by coronary artery disease or idiopathic myocardial disease (e.g. cardiomyopathy) will result in ECG changes. ECG abnormalities in cardiomyopathy are often non-diagnostic while in coronary artery disease they are quite characteristic and diagnostic, particularly in the acute phase. ECG abnormalities include ST depression for chronic ischaemia, ST elevation for acute myocardial infarction and pathological Q waves for old myocardial infarction. The location of such abnormalities among the 12 ECG leads is suggestive of the coronary territories (table 16.1 and figure 16-1).

Ischaemia location	ECG leads	Coronary territory
Anteroseptal	V1, V2 and V3	Proximal LAD
Extensive anterior	V1 to V4 (V5 or V6)	LAD and Cx
Lateral	V5 and V6, I and avL	Cx
Inferior	II, III and avF	RCA, occasionally Cx
Posterior	Mirror images of V1, V2 and V3	Cx
Note: Cx – circumflex coronary artery; **LAD** – left anterior descending coronary artery; **RCA** – right coronary artery		

Table 16-1 Relation of ischaemia on ECG and coronary artery territory

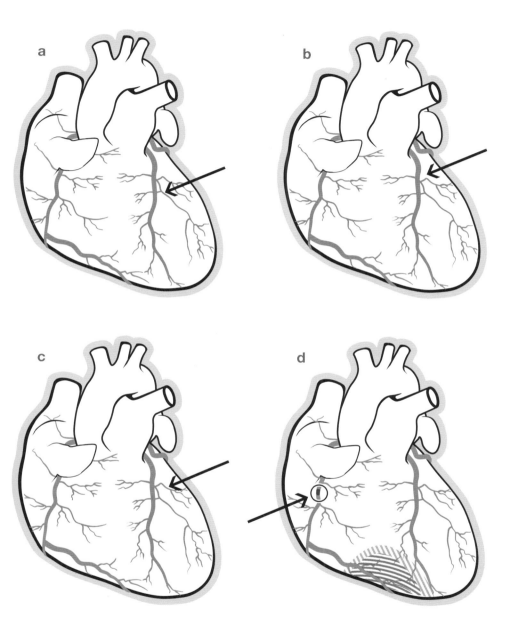

Figure 16-1 a-d Correlation between localisation of infarction and occlusion of coronary artery (arrow)
a. Anteroseptal infarction   **c.** Isolated lateral infarction
b. Extensive anterior infarction   **d.** Inferior infarction

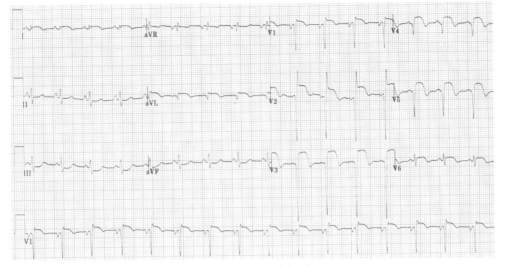

Figure 16-2 An ECG example of acute ST elevation myocardial infarction

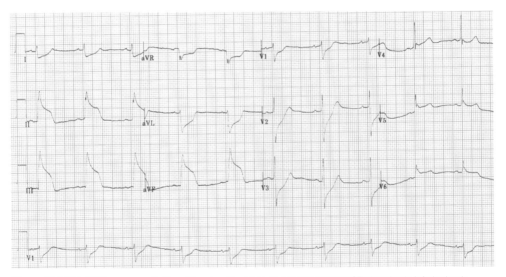

Figure 16-3 This ECG was recorded in a 63-year-old woman and shows obvious ST elevation in inferior leads, V5 and V6, and ST depression in V1 to V3 (reciprocal changes). This is a typical example of acute inferior myocardial infarction

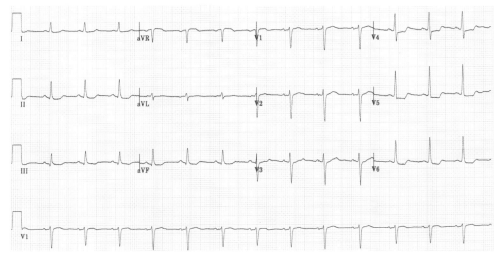

Figure 16-4 This ECG was recorded in a 78-year-old woman who presented in A & E with typical chest pain, normal troponin and CK. There is no typical ST elevation but ST depression. She was managed as unstable angina

Acute myocardial infarction

Case history

A 52-year-old Asian man was admitted to CCU with a history of two hours of crushing chest pain and dyspnoea. The patient was very unwell on examination.

ECG findings

This shows sinus rhythm with a heart rate of 100 bpm. The PR interval, QRS duration, QRS axis and QT interval are all normal. There is ST elevation across all chest leads and, less obviously, in leads I and avL. There were also Q waves in the same leads (figure 16-2).

ECG diagnosis: acute extensive anterior myocardial infarction, probably on top of old myocardial infarction.

ECG diagnostic criteria for acute myocardial infarction: the main feature of acute myocardial infarction is ST elevation. The location of ST elevation on the ECG can be a good indicator to the culprit coronary arteries (table 1).

Comments

Acute myocardial infarction is still associated with high mortality, particularly in those who are unable to reach hospitals within the first hour. ECG is usually the first and most likely available test. ST elevation is characteristic and often diagnostic. The location of ischaemia and responsible coronary arteries can be defined by the affected ECG leads (figure 16-3). However, not all acute myocardial infarction presents with ST elevation that is referred to as non-ST elevation myocardial infarction, of which the clinical presentation can be similar to ST elevation myocardial infarction (figure 16-2 and 16-3) or unstable angina (figure 16-4).

What to do next

Prompt thrombolysis or coronary intervention is the key treatment for acute myocardial infarction. This patient was admitted to CCU and started on thrombolytic therapy. He should also have immediate risk factor stratification.

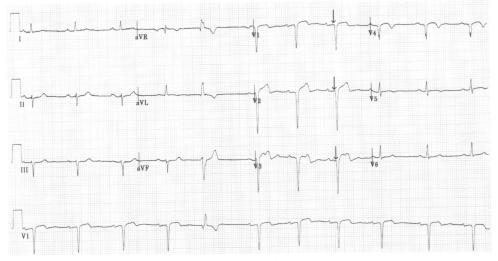

Figure 16-5 An ECG example of old anterior myocardial infarction

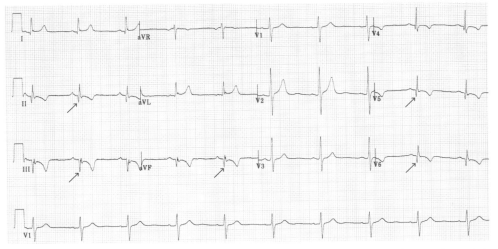

Figure 16-6 This ECG is an example of old lateral and inferior myocardial infarction (Q waves by arrows) recorded in a 77-year-old woman

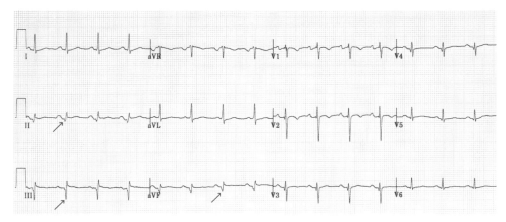

Figure 16-7 This ECG is an example of old inferior myocardial infarction (Q waves by arrows) recorded in a 60-year-old man

Old myocardial infarction

Case history

A 67-year-old woman had been treated for an acute myocardial infarction a year previously. She was under cardiology follow-up.

ECG findings

This shows sinus rhythm with a heart rate of 72 bpm. The PR interval, QRS duration, QRS axis and QT interval are all normal. There are Q waves (arrows) in leads V1, V2 and V3 (figure 16-5).

ECG diagnosis: old anterior myocardial infarction.

ECG diagnostic criteria for old myocardial infarction: the characteristic feature for old myocardial infarction is pathological Q waves. A pathological Q wave is a Q wave wider than 40 ms (one small square) in duration and taller than ¼ of the QRS amplitude. The location of the Q waves on the body surface ECG is used to define the culprit coronary arteries (table 16-1).

Comments

Clinical management of old myocardial infarction depends upon its size and location. Extensive anterior myocardial infarction is usually associated with left ventricular failure and poor prognosis. Revascularisation should be actively considered in all cases.

There are some more ECG examples of old myocardial infarction in relation to coronary territory (figures 16-6 to 16-8).

What to do next

In all patients with old myocardial infarction, risk factor stratification including treating co-existing risk factors and lifestyle modification is the corner stone.

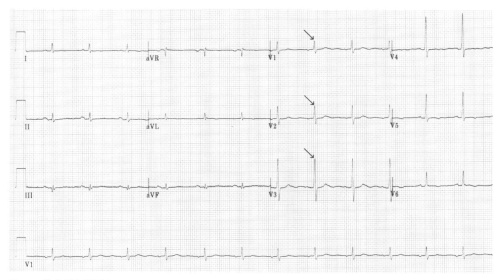

Figure 16-8 This ECG is an example of old posterior myocardial infarction (R waves in V1 to V3 by arrows are equivalent to Q waves from the posterior wall) recorded in a 78-year-old woman

17 ACUTE PERICARDITIS

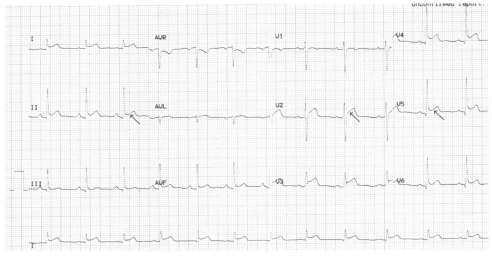

Figure 17-1 An ECG example of acute pericarditis

Acute pericarditis

Case history

A 19-year-old man had been recently admitted to hospital because of chest pain and was generally unwell. An echocardiogram showed slightly impaired left ventricular function but no obvious pericardial effusion.

ECG findings

This shows sinus rhythm with a heart rate of 95 bpm. The QRS axis is normal, so are PR interval, QRS duration and QT interval. QRS amplitude is normal with no beat-to-beat variation. There is, however, ST elevation in most ECG leads (arrows, figure 17.1).

ECG diagnosis: pericarditis.

ECG diagnostic criteria for pericarditis: the main ECG feature is "concave-upwards" ST elevation.

Other ECG changes associated with pericarditis include sinus tachycardia, reduced QRS voltage or electrical alternans, i.e. alternating short and tall QRS complexes (see page 106, figure 20-4) if there is a large pericardial effusion.

Comments

This ECG shows the typical concave ST elevation of acute pericarditis with a slightly increased heart rate. Attention needs to be paid to the differentiation of ST elevation in other conditions including acute myocardial infarction.

What to do next

Patients with acute pericarditis should be hospitalised for appropriate investigation and treatment. In particular, observations should include the development of pericardial effusion by echocardiography.

18 EXERCISE STRESS ECG

Exercise stress ECG is used for both hospital and primary care patients. Most GP-led exercise ECG testing is conducted, for example, in rapid access chest pain clinics. It provides information on the diagnosis of coronary artery disease in patients with exertional symptoms, patients with atypical symptoms and female patients with chest pain both typical and atypical. It can help perform the assessment of functional capacity in patients with stable angina or after myocardial infarction or patients with valvular disease. It can also help assess the prognosis in patients with angiographically confirmed coronary artery disease, patients having recovered from acute myocardial infarction or those treated for heart failure.

LEARNING POINTS

1   Exercise is commonly used to diagnose coronary artery disease.

2   It is less reliable in women because of the higher incidence of false positive results.

The most commonly used method for an exercise stress ECG test is the standard Bruce treadmill protocol. In this protocol, the treadmill starts at a 1.7 mph speed and 10% slope (5 METs) with an increase in both speed and slope every three minutes (Stage) up to 5.0 mph and 18% respectively. In older patients or those whose exercise capacity is limited, the Bruce protocol can be modified by two 3-minute warm-up stages at 1.7 mph and 0% slope.

However, the exercise stress test should not be used in patients with:

- ongoing acute myocardial ischaemia
- unstable angina.
- very high blood pressure, systolic pressure ≥230 mmHg or diastolic pressure ≥110 mmHg
- myocarditis
- pericarditis
- severe aortic stenosis
- any acute systemic illness.

Some other conditions, though not contraindicated for the test, are difficult to interpret or not suitable for exercise stress:

- complete right bundle branch block
- atrial fibrillation
- baseline ST-T abnormalities
- chronic obstructive airways disease
- severe obesity
- peripheral vascular disease
- arthritis
- any inability of walking on a treadmill regardless of cause.

Patients with such conditions could have alternative approaches to the investigation of inducible myocardial ischaemia, such as nuclear imaging and stress echocardiography.

There are small chances of risks associated with an exercise stress test. For instance, exercise provoked myocardial infarction or life-threatening arrhythmias are reported in up to five out of 10 000 (0.05%) tests, and death in up to one out of 10 000 (0.01%).

During an exercise stress test, heart rate and blood pressure increase, PR interval and QRS duration may both shorten, QRS complex and T wave amplitude may reduce slightly. The main features of a positive exercise test include (figure 18-1):

- horizontal or downsloping ST depression over 1.5 mm
- upsloping ST depression over 1.5 mm that does not recover back to baseline at 80 ms.

Despite its limitations, coronary angiography is still widely accepted as the gold standard for the diagnosis of coronary artery disease. Using coronary angiography as a standard, an exercise stress test has an overall 70% sensitivity and specificity. In single vessel disease, it has a mean sensitivity of 68% (23 - 100%) and a mean specificity of 77% (17 - 100%). In two-vessel disease, it has a mean sensitivity of 81% (40 - 100%) and a mean specificity of 66% (17 - 100%). In triple-vessel disease or left anterior descending coronary artery lesion, it has the highest sensitivity (86±11%) but lowest specificity (53±24%). However, one must bear in mind that there are differences between men and women in an exercise test. False positive results are more common in women than in men and reduce the diagnostic accuracy in women.

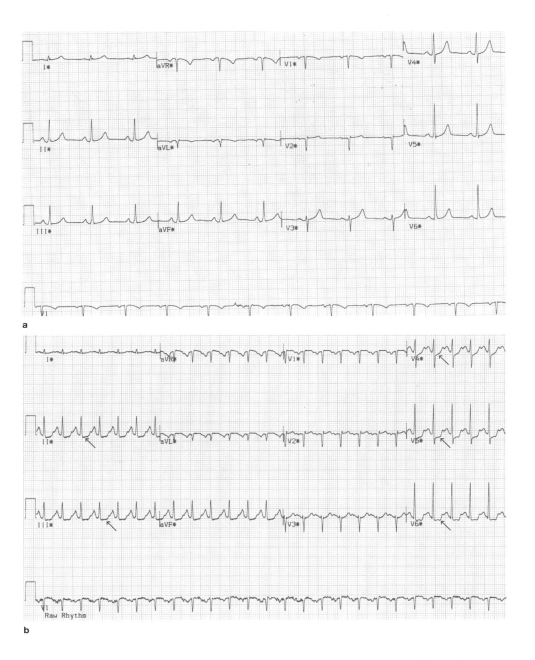

Figure 18-1 An exercise stress ECG test was performed in a 62-year-old woman with atypical chest pain. The resting ECG (a) shows nearly diminished R wave in V1 and V2 but no ST-T changes. After 7 minutes on the Bruce Protocol, she achieved 100% maximum predicted heart rate (158 bpm) and became significantly breathless. The ECG at peak stress (b) shows horizontal ST depression in inferior and lateral leads (arrows). This is a positive exercise ECG indicating inducible ischaemia

19 PACING ECGs

Patients with advanced heart block require a pacemaker to maintain their heart beats and thus circulation. More recently pacemakers have been used to treat advanced heart failure for functional improvement. It is practically important to recognise a pacing ECG and even work out the type of pacemaker from the body surface ECG. The key to pacing ECG interpretation is to identify the pacing spike (artificial stimulation) which, as in spontaneous cardiac excitation, is followed by depolarisation and repolarisation. The following are the most common types of pacing ECGs.

LEARNING POINTS

---

1 A pacemaker is traditionally used to treat high degree heart block, though it has been recently used to improve cardiac function in advanced heart failure.

2 The key to pacing ECGs is to identify the simulation spike.

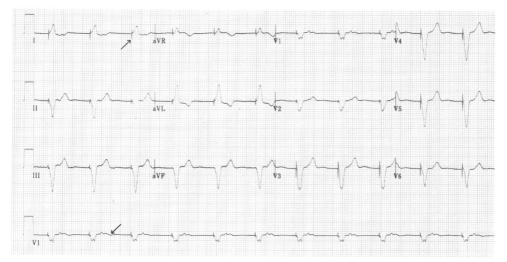

Figure 19-1 An ECG example of VVI pacing. There are pacing spikes (blue arrow) followed by a QRS complex and P waves after the QRS complex (black arrow) defined as retrograde conducted P waves

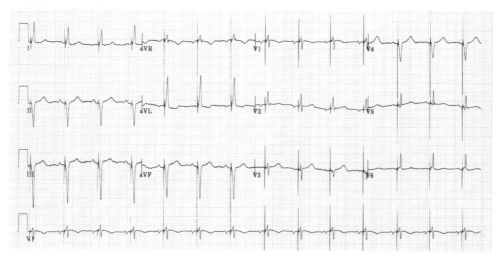

Figure 19-2 An ECG example of DDD pacing. Pacing spikes for both atrium and ventricle divided in constant time interval (AV delay) and followed by a P wave and a QRS complex, respectively

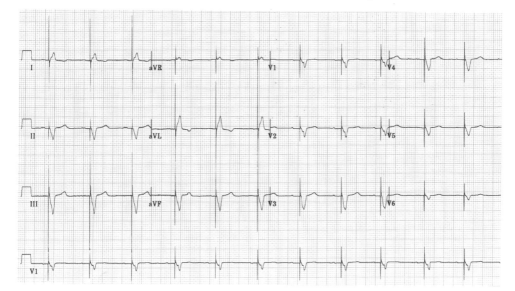

Figure 19-3 Another ECG example of DDD pacing with the atrial pacing spike after the P wave and before the QRS complex

20 UNCOMMON ECGs

Apart from the common abnormal ECGs, there are a variety of less common ones. It is very important to recognise these uncommon ECG patterns, particularly when making differential diagnoses and predicting the prognosis.

LEARNING POINTS

1 It is equally important to recognise some rare ECG abnormalities .

2 In this section, we include long QT syndrome, Brugada syndrome, dextracardia, electrical alternan and abnormal U wave.

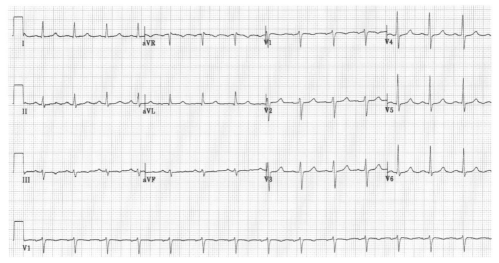

Figure 20-1 An ECG example of long QT syndrome

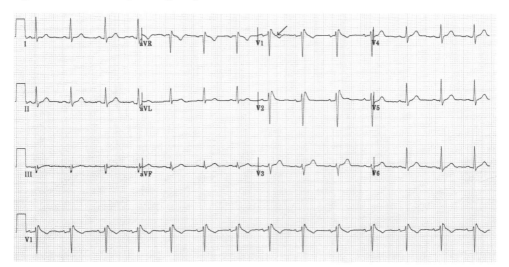

Figure 20-2 An ECG example of Brugada syndrome

Long QT syndrome

The ECG is the only reliable diagnostic tool for long QT syndrome (figure 20-1) (the corrected QT interval over 450 ms). Regardless of aetiology, long QT interval can be associated with early cardiac death.

Brugada syndrome

Brugada syndrome (figure 20-2) is characterised by RSR pattern in leads V1 and V2 (similar to right bundle branch block) and ST elevation (arrow), which can be easily taken as acute anterior myocardial infarction. Brugada syndrome is a rare condition and may result in sudden death.

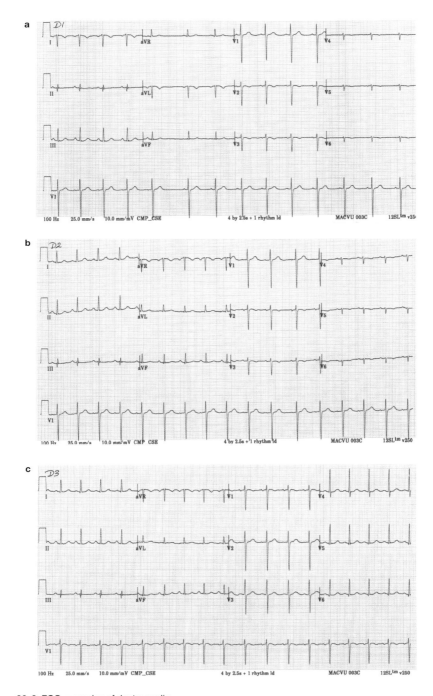

Figure 20-3 ECG examples of dextracardia

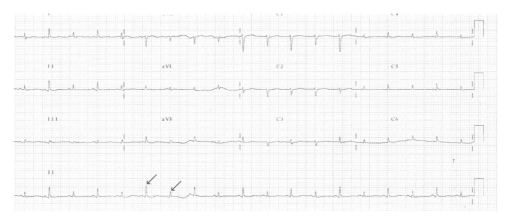

Figure 20-4 An ECG example of electrical alternan

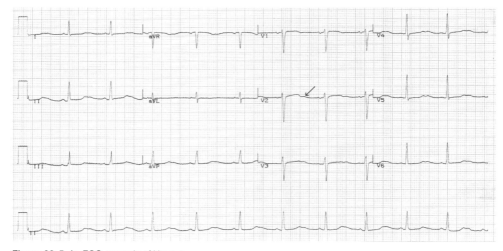

Figure 20-5 An ECG example of U wave

Dextracardia

In patients with dextracadia, the ECG is a mirror image of the normal as is the heart itself. With the normal ECG lead placement, the significant right axis deviation (big S wave in lead I and big R wave in lead III), and QRS amplitude decreases from the right to the left chest leads (figure 20-3a). When the limb leads are reversed, the QRS axis becomes normal (figure 20-3b) and when, in addition, the chest leads are also reversed, the whole ECG becomes normal (figure 20-3 c).

Electrical alternan

This is characterised by the change in QRS amplitude (arrows, figure 20-4). This is the ECG sign of big pericardial collection resulting in cardiac tamponade.

Prominent U wave

A prominent U wave (arrow, figure 20-5) is an ECG manifestation of hypokalemia. This ECG was recorded in a patient with a serum potassium level of 2.7 mmol/L.

21 HOW TO CHOOSE AN ECG MACHINE

In order to buy an adequate ECG machine, one must avoid just browsing brochures or websites and assuming equal quality of all products. There are a wide range of ECG recorders available in the market but, unfortunately, the technical specifications are either missing from the glossy brochures and websites or difficult to understand. It is, however, very important to request and probably familiarise yourself with the basic technical specifications to make sure they meet the minimum recommendations before a purchase is made.

It is well recognised that ECG interpretation depends on the recording quality which is principally determined by the appropriate technical specifications of the ECG recorder. There have been comprehensive recommendations in the literature [1-4] and readers could refer to them for detailed information. In this chapter, we only summarise the minimum recommendations for the main technical specifications (also see table 21-1).

LEARNING POINTS

---

1   The two most important technical parameters for an ECG machine are frequency response and sampling rate.

Parameter	Recommendation
Frequency response	0.05 – 100 Hz (0.05 – 250 Hz for young children)
Time accuracy	<5 ms
Amplitude accuracy	<20 uV
Gain settings	5 mm/mV, 10 mm/mV and 20 mm/mV
Chart speed for print-out	25 mm/sec or 50 mm/sec
Trace width for print-out	<1 mm
Sampling rate	500 Hz/lead

Table 21-1 Recommended minimum requirements for an ECG machine

Frequency response

This is the ability of an ECG recorder to register the frequency spectrum of input signals. The frequency of the myocardial electric current ranges mostly from 0.05 to 100 Hz in adults, and up to 250 Hz in children. An ECG recorder with adequate quality should be able to register signals from 0.05 to 150 Hz in frequency. The high frequency response helps ECG recorders register high frequency signals, such as small R waves. On the contrary, low frequency response helps to keep the fidelity of the low frequency signals, such as ST shift and T waves. It is therefore very important to bear in mind that inadequate high frequency response leads to serious distortion of the QRS complex and inadequate low frequency response leads to serious distortion of the ST segment and T wave.

Signal fidelity and sampling rate

The closeness of the recorded traces to the original signals is fidelity, which can be illustrated in amplitude and time. An adequate quality ECG recorder should be able to record signals ≤ 20 uV in amplitude and ≤ 5ms in duration. For print-out ECG traces, there should be gain controls of 10 mm/1 mV, 5 mm/1 mV and 20 mm/1 mV for amplitude. The time sensitivity of modern ECG recorders is largely determined by the speed of original signals being acquired, the sampling rate. The minimum recommended sampling rate is 500 Hz per lead. Thus, an ECG recorder must have a sampling rate of 6 KHz to record a 12-lead ECG. The ECG traces are usually printed out at a paper speed of 25 mm/s.

The purchase of an ECG recorder is a reasonably valuable investment if it meets the minimum technical recommendations. Like any other investment, one should try to understand the nature of the product, and probably seek professional advice should there be any uncertainty.

Further reading:

1 Bailey JJ, Berson AS, Garson A Jr, Horan LG, Macfarlane PW, Mortara DW, Zywietz C. Recommendations for standardization and specifications in automated electrocardiography: bandwidth and digital signal processing. A report for health professionals by an ad hoc writing group of the Committee on Electrocardiography and Cardiac Electrophysiology of the Council on Clinical Cardiology, American Heart Association. *Circulation* 1990; **81**:730-9.

2 Pipberger HV. The "new" electrocardiographs. A step toward greater fidelity in recording (editorial). *Circulation* 1970;**52**;771-2.

3 Kossmann CE, Broday D, Burch GE *et al.* Recommendations for standardization of leads and of specifications for instruments in electrocardiography and vectocardiography. Report of the Committee on Electrocardiography, American Heart Association. *Circulation* 1967; **35**:583-602.

4 Pipberger HV, Arzbaecher RC, Berson AS *et al.* Recommendations for standardization and specifications for instruments in electrocardiography vectocardiography. Report of the Committee on Electrocardiography, American Heart Association. *Circulation* 1975; **52**:11-33.

PART 3

INDEX

PRESCRIBING INFORMATION

ADULT ADVANCED LIFE SUPPORT ALGORITHM

INDEX

PLAVIX®

Prescribing Information

Presentation: Round, pink, film coated tablets containing 75mg clopidogrel (as the bisulphate).

Indication: Reduction of atherothrombotic events in patients with a history of symptomatic atherosclerotic disease defined by ischaemic stroke (from 7 days until less than 6 months), myocardial infarction (from a few days until less than 35 days) or established peripheral arterial disease; in combination with aspirin, in patients with unstable angina (UA) or non-ST-elevation MI (NSTEMI); in combination with aspirin in patients with ST elevation MI (STEMI) eligible for fibrinolytic therapy.

Dosage: Adults and elderly: 75mg as a single daily dose. In patients with UA/NSTEMI: single 300mg loading dose, followed by 75mg daily (with aspirin 75-100mg/day); clinical trial data support use up to 12 months (maximum benefit at 3 months). In patients with STEMI: a loading dose in those aged less than 75 years followed by 75mg daily in combination with aspirin, with or without thrombolytics, started as early as possible and continued for at least 4 weeks (beyond 4 weeks has not been studied). No loading dose is required in patients aged greater than 75 years. Children and adolescents: Not recommended under 18 years.

Contraindications: Hypersensitivity to clopidogrel or excipients; severe liver impairment; active pathological bleeding; breast-feeding.

Warnings: Due to the risk of bleeding and haematological disorders, blood cell count determination should be conducted where suspected clinical symptoms suggestive of bleeding arise during treatment; monitor for signs of bleeding, especially during the first weeks of treatment and after invasive cardiac procedures or surgery; caution in patients with lesions likely to bleed, particularly gastrointestinal and intraocular; renal impairment; hepatic disease. Discontinue therapy 7 days prior to surgery. Not recommended during pregnancy.

Drug Interactions: Not recommended with warfarin. Caution when used with aspirin (although combination used together for up to one year in the CURE study), NSAIDs (including COX 2 inhibitors), heparin, thrombolytics, glycoprotein IIb/IIIa inhibitors.

Side Effects: Haematological disorders: very rare cases of thrombotic thrombocytopenic purpura, severe thrombocytopenia, neutropenia, agranulocytosis, anaemia and aplastic anaemia / pancytopenia; Haemorrhagic disorders: serious bleeding such as skin bleeding, bruising, haemarthrosis, haematoma, eye bleeding, epistaxis, respiratory tract bleeding, haematuria and intracranial, gastrointestinal and retroperitoneal haemorrhage and haemorrhage of operative wound. Significantly increased risk of major/minor bleeding when used with aspirin (dose dependent); Gastrointestinal disorders: diarrhoea, very rare reports of colitis, pancreatitis and stomatitis; Urinary/hepatic disorders: very rare cases of renal disorders, abnormal creatinine levels, abnormal liver function tests, hepatitis and acute liver failure; Allergic disorders: very rare skin reactions, angioedema, anaphylactoid reactions and serum sickness; Musculoskeletal disorders; very rare reports of arthralgia, arthritis and myalgia; Others: very rare cases of taste disorders, confusion, hallucinations, fever, vasculitis, hypotension, bronchospasm and interstitial pneumonitis. Please consult SPC for full details of the recognised side effects with Plavix.

Legal category: POM

Product Licence Number: EU/1/98/069/001a

Marketing authorisation Holder:
Sanofi Pharma Bristol-Myers Squibb SNC

Further information is available from: sanofi-aventis, One Onslow Street, Guildford, Surrey, GU1 4YS Tel: 01483 505515 Fax: 01483 535432

Basic NHS Price: £35.31 for 28 tablets

Date of preparation: September 2006

® denotes a Registered Trade Mark.

Information about adverse event reporting can be found on www.yellowcard.gov.uk

Adverse events should also be reported to the sanofi-aventis Drug Safety Department.

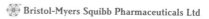

Adult advanced life support algorithm

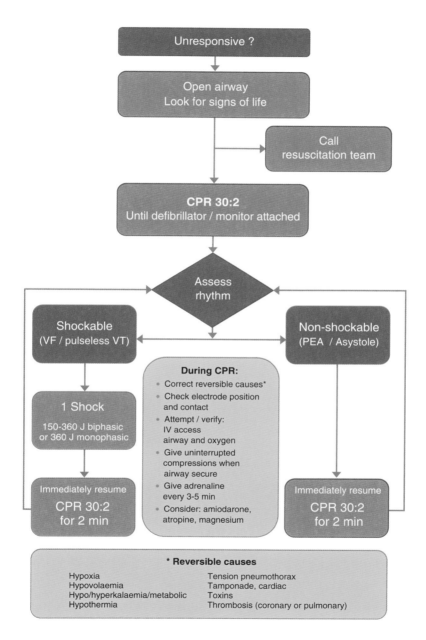

CPR = cardiopulmonary resuscitation